PAIN AND ITS CONQUEST

PAIN

AND ITS CONQUEST

H. B. GIBSON

PETER OWEN · LONDON AND BOSTON

ISBN 0 7206 0595 4

PETER OWEN PUBLISHERS
73 Kenway Road London SW5 0RE
and 99 Main Street Salem NH 03079

First published 1982
© H. B. Gibson 1982

Printed in Great Britain by
Photobooks (Bristol) Ltd
Barton Manor, St. Philips, Bristol

To all my colleagues
in the International Association
for the Study of Pain

CONTENTS

ACKNOWLEDGEMENTS

In writing this book I have been indebted to a large number of people, many of them members of the International Association for the Study of Pain (IASP), who have given me their time in discussions and in correspondence. I should like particularly to mention Dr D. L. Scott (Whiston Hospital, Cheshire), who advised me regarding modern methods of anaesthesia. Dr W. C. Coe (California State University, Fresno) was good enough to clarify his position regarding the controversial matter of the inhibition of pain by hypnosis, and I have quoted him verbatim in Chapter 5. A draft of that chapter was read and commented on by both Professor L. Chertok (Centre de Médicine Psychosomatique, Paris) and Professor E. R. Hilgard (Stanford University).

Professor H. J. Eysenck (Institute of Psychiatry, London) and Professor L. Von Knorring (Umeä University, Sweden) read a draft of the more controversial part of Chapter 6 which concerns their work and commented on it. Dr Asenath Petrie (Jerusalem) advised regarding some aspects of her work mentioned in Chapter 6. Professor J. J. Bonica (University of Washington) and Professor D. Albe-Fessard (Université Pierre et Marie Curie, Paris) kindly agreed to the reproduction of the list of speciality areas of the IASP in Appendix 1; it originally appeared in *Advances in Pain Research and Therapy* (1976), published by Raven Press, New York, to whom acknowledgement is also made. Dr R. Melzack (McGill University) kindly sent me a copy of his McGill-Melzack Pain Questionnaire, which is reproduced in Appendix 2. I am also indebted to Dr Clare Phillips and Dr Jane Wardle (both of the Institute of Psychiatry, London) for sending me so much material, published and unpublished, relating to recent developments in pain research.

Finally, I must acknowledge my debt to a number of past patients for their most insightful comments on their conditions of pain and on the measures taken to alleviate it. They are the ones who know where the shoe pinches, and without their commentaries on experience and treatment we investigators and theoreticians could make little progress in our research.

H.B.G.

INTRODUCTION

This book is intended as both a theoretical elucidation of the phenomenon of pain, and as a practical manual addressed to those who suffer pain and also to those who in their professional and private capacities seek to understand and alleviate it. It is written from the point of view of a psychologist and is particularly concerned with psychological methods of controlling pain, but it also aims to take account of the neurological, physiological and philosophical problems involved.

There are several reasons for writing such a book at this time. We have recently entered a new era in which previous concepts about the nature of pain, and views concerning the appropriateness of some existing forms of treatment, have undergone quite rapid changes and development, due to research findings in a number of related disciplines. No longer can the medical practitioner depend entirely on the simple statements about pain given in the standard textbooks which he used as a medical student, or accept uncritically views about the treatment of pain which are implied on the voluminous literature issued by the drug companies. Essentially, the future lies with interdisciplinary collaboration; the founding, in 1974, of the International Association for the Study of Pain (see Appendix 1) attests to the wide range of professional disciplines involved. For those who, a few years ago, expected that they, or members of their families, were doomed to suffer years of racking pain with all its personal and social consequences, and for medical practitioners frustrated by the failure of their humane endeavours to control pain, the new approaches considered in this book offer fresh hope.

The greatest battle in the campaign for the conquest of pain has already been won. With the sudden introduction of anaesthetics in medicine and dentistry in the mid nineteenth century came changes in old *attitudes* to pain, although these lingered on for some time in the field of obstetrics. In fact, as we shall see, the great technical innovation of anaesthesia could have occurred half a century before it did; the reasons for this delay can be traced to earlier attitudes to pain shared by both patients and the majority of physicians and nurses. With the acceptance of pain-free surgery as a right, the role of pain in general sickness was seen in an altered light, and there was a general growth in compassion, a compassion that has spread, and is spreading, into areas of social life beyond the hospital and sick-room.

The 'gate control' theory of pain, first postulated in the 1960s by Melzack and Wall, has had a powerful effect on the conceptualization of pain and on the development of research into its problems. The complexity of many of the areas in which Melzack and Wall were working precludes a full exposition of this fertile theory in a book intended to be comprehensible throughout to the educated layman, but it will be apparent that the views of the author have been strongly influenced by its sophisticated marrying of psychological with neurological theory. The way of regarding pain that we all grow up with is bound by the simple 'push-button' theory of pain, as Melzack has termed it. This simple and traditional theory is of course tacitly accepted by most general practitioners, hospital consultants, dentists, physiotherapists and others who deal with pain. It is, however, somewhat inadequate to deal with the difficult problems of chronic pain and so-called 'psychogenic' pain. The chapters devoted to a discussion of the nature of pain and its relations with the emotions and mechanisms of perception will consider this point.

As the orientation of this study is psychological, a good deal of attention has been paid to the control of pain by hypnosis. This may surprise some readers, for the subject of hypnosis is still surrounded by myth and superstition, and it has yet to be generally accepted as a psychological phenomenon that can be studied scientifically and employed to great effect in therapy. Indeed, no adequate discussion of the historical development of anaesthesia, in its widest sense, or of modern methods of the psychological control of pain, can omit some history of mesmerism and the development of hypnotism as it is currently understood.

In dealing with problems in which pain may arise, general practitioners may, to some extent, be divided between those who think in terms of 'conditions' and those who think in terms of 'people'. Ordinary practice may teach that certain conditions are painful and that others are not. But there are always anomalies: some 'non-painful' conditions (including those in which there appears to be nothing organically wrong) are accompanied in some patients by persistent complaints of pain. To silence such complaints, huge quantities of pills are regularly prescribed, not just to the complainers but as a sop to the pill-hungry public at large. A relatively undeveloped area of pain research is relevant to this problem, that of individual differences in susceptibility to pain. These differences are very real, and demonstrate that it is entirely artificial to think of pathological conditions in themselves as 'painful' or 'non-painful'. It is the people who need to be studied with respect to their pain, and there is much truth in the old adage which holds that only the wearer knows where the shoe pinches.

The problem of individual differences in susceptibility to pain has been approached in two ways. First, by psychiatrists using clinical judgement and a widely-known psychiatric questionnaire known as the Minnesota Multiphasic Personality Inventory (MMPI); but their research has been somewhat biased by the fact that it has chiefly been confined to psychiatric populations, whereas the main problem concerns the public at large. The second approach has concentrated on the normal population, and much of it has concerned the infliction of experimental pain on subjects who have been induced to volunteer for such laboratory research. In its early days this type of work came in for a great deal of criticism from those who pointed out that pain inflicted in the laboratory and pain encountered in the surgery, clinic and hospital differ in many important respects, which may lead to false conclusions being drawn. Foremost among the critics was Professor Beecher, one of the greatest of the early pioneers of pain research, and his immense prestige delayed the development of laboratory research. Eventually Beecher came round to acknowledging the relevance of research into experimental pain, and it is now a fruitful field of research, well integrated with clinical studies.

This field of laboratory research into experimentally induced pain has included a great deal of fundamental research into measurable differences in personality, such as that stemming from Eysenck and his associates, notably that of Asenath Petrie whose early work, while controversial, still continues to have a seminal influence in many laboratories.

A special chapter has been devoted to 'women's pains', for they exemplify the remarkable fact that for one half of the population, normal physiological functions involve the potentiality of pain. The feminist movement has drawn attention to the fact that many of the pains which are specific to the female sex have tended to be treated rather cavalierly by the medical profession, and has related this to the tradition of male dominance in that profession. The study of women's pains, notably those of childbirth, has been a special issue at different historical times, and has thrown light on the relationship between pain in general and social attitudes. For example, when anaesthesia first became generally available, there was some debate as to whether artificial aid should be granted to minimize the pain of childbirth; it was maintained by some physicians and churchmen that this was a 'natural' pain. Half a century later, there was optimism that pain in childbirth might in any case be *unnecessary*, as it may result entirely from unnatural attitudes engendered by our modern way of living.

The hopes of such pioneers as Grantly Dick Read and the Russian school of Psychoprophylaxis that pain in childbirth could be totally eliminated have not been fulfilled, but their partial fulfilment has certainly revolutionized obstetric care, and waves of feminist protest keep the problem in the foreground. The fact is, as we shall see, that the mechanisms of pain in childbirth are still incompletely understood; it is a mystery why a minority of women, who do not appear to have any special anatomical or other peculiarity, experience virtually no pain in childbirth. This poses problems of immense importance for the whole field of pain research.

Arising out of the study of obstetric pain, and out of other areas of pain research, an approach is suggested in this book, the Epicurean approach, which brings in a psychological perspective contrasting the Stoic with the Epicurean philosophy, and which may have very practical applications not only in therapy for pain, but also in the development of personality adjustments which better enable us to come to terms with conditions which are potentially productive of pain.

Although the first phase in the campaign for the conquest of pain has been virtually won by the spectacular success of medical science in anaesthesia, we are left with the problems of chronic pain. These problems, which are now the main subject of research and therapy, of course increase in a population which is steadily becoming over-weighted with the elderly. Each one of us has to confront the question: How shall we live out whatever we consider should be the natural span of our lives without becoming a burden to ourselves, our families and the caring professions because of the many painful conditions which attend the natural decay of our bodies? Here, what is being learnt in the rehabilitation of those who suffer from chronically painful conditions resulting from injuries and diseases earlier in life, has much to offer in developing techniques for assisting the elderly. It is suggested that the Epicurean approach is relevant to this therapy. The role of psychologists in treatment and research has undoubtedly been increased by the extended study of chronic pain, and here perhaps this book has most to offer. It is the intimate personal concern of every member of the community, even though at present he may be in perfect health, for none of us can afford to neglect John Donne's warning:

Never send to know for whom the bell tolls: it tolls for thee.

1

HISTORICAL BACKGROUND

Ancient Anodynes

All cultures throughout history have endeavoured to banish pain, and their literature and mythologies include records of the various methods employed to accomplish this humane end. The first surgical operation performed on man, and performed painlessly by reason of an induced sleep, is that described in Genesis 2: 21: 'And the Lord God caused a deep sleep to fall on Adam, and he slept: and He took one of his ribs and closed up the flesh instead thereof.'

In ancient literature sleep is often mentioned as the means whereby pain is prevented, but sometimes anodynes, or analgesics as we would now call them, are referred to. In the *Iliad* Patroclus comes to the aid of the wounded Eurypylus before Troy. After cutting an arrow-shaft from his thigh, he

> Then pounded in his hands, the root applied
> Astringent, anodyne, which all his pain
> Allay'd; the wound was dried and staunched the blood.[1]

Before proceeding further, we must discriminate between the meanings of two words used repeatedly in the discussion of pain: 'anaesthesia' and 'analgesia'. Anaesthesia signifies a total loss of sensation. Thus a person who is unconscious by reason of being anaesthetized by a drug, will show little or no reaction to stimuli which are normally painful, nor will he report any memory of being hurt. This is known as 'general' anaesthesia. In practice, surgical operations are not always conducted with the patient in the very deepest state of anaesthesia, and, although the patient does not suffer, some residual sensation may be present. Patients under general anaesthesia have even been shown to have some memory of conversations that have taken place in the operating theatre.[2] In 'local' anaesthesia, a specific area of the body is rendered without feeling by, for instance, the injection of a drug like novacaine, for the purpose of a minor operation.

'Analgesia' does not mean total loss of sensation, but loss of the experience of pain. Thus an aching rheumatic limb may be eased by an analgesic drug like aspirin. The limb does not became anaesthetic; it remains perfectly sensitive to touch, heat and cold, but the ache is abolished. All anaesthetics are of course analgesics, because if total sensation is removed there is no pain.

In the Homeric epics the word *pharmakon* is used to mean either a drug or a charm, and it is this dual method of treating pain, the pharmacological and the psychological, which has caused confusion right up until the present day. All drugs have some magical (psychological) associations, and their action does not depend on their chemical properties alone. Factors such as the observance of a proper ritual, the favour of a god, the healing intent of the therapist and the faith of the patient may play as important a part as the chemical nature of the drug. Indeed, sometimes all resort to physical medicine is dispensed with, and pain and sickness are overcome by entirely psychological means, as in the ancient practices of *Chuff* and *Jar Phoonk*, or the mesmerism of the eighteenth and nineteenth centuries.

While fully acknowledging the need to respect ritualistic observances, and dedicating their temples of healing to the god Asclepius, the Greek doctors from about the time of Hippocrates (400 BC) assiduously sought to discover the pharmacological properties of the plants they used in medicine. The chief pain-killers were mandragora (from the mandrake), opium poppy, Indian hemp, dittany, hemlock, henbane and, especially, wine. The role of wine in analgesia and anaesthesia was all important, and whatever plants and other substances were employed in the ancient recipes, they were generally administered in wine. An individual specimen of any plant may contain a widely varying quantity of the active principle, and so, lacking the means to assess the strength of any brew prepared, the physician might well kill his patient by administering too potent a concoction. It became the practice, therefore, to err on the side of caution by mixing a small quantity of the plant juices with a much larger quantity of strong wine. Thus the patient's pain was safely allayed by Bacchus if not by Asclepius.

Alcohol is indeed one of the most benign drugs, for unlike those derived from many of the classic medicinal plants, it will seldom cause sudden death. It operates principally not by dulling the senses and thus overcoming pain by narcosis, but by acting as a euphoriant and elevating the mood, so that strong sensations previously experienced as pain may be tolerated with equanimity.

It is of interest that the Greeks, innovating scientists though they were, still attributed a special wisdom to the older civilization of

Egypt. Pliny states that the Egyptian physicians used a powdered rock, obtained from Memphis, which, when moistened with vinegar, would assuage the pain of wounds. If this is true, as suggested by Kleiman,[3] it is the first recorded use of carbonic acid gas as a local anaesthetic. Medicine was certainly well advanced in Egypt in ancient times, and the George Ebers papyrus discovered in the Theban Acropolis lists 700 medical remedies, including the opium poppy. But although many of them indicate that much empirical research had been conducted, there were also such strange remedies as 'water in which the phallus has been washed'. The Egyptians also experimented with the inhalation of fumes to produce sleep and anaesthesia. The fumes produced by heating Indian hemp (*cannabis indica*) – bringing on in those who breathe them a state of mental exaltation, sometimes followed by sleep – were widely used as an analgesic in the Middle East, although their effects were uncertain.

The ancient Jews also recorded various remedies for pain, and it is notable that they showed a compassion for the suffering of condemned criminals. The 'potion of the condemned' was a stupefying drink, probably containing mandragora, which produced a dulling of pain and perhaps an early death in criminals suffering execution. The potion which was offered on a sponge to Christ on the cross is variously described in the gospels as wine or vinegar mixed with gall, myrrh or hyssop.[4]

The Magical Mandrake

Although the juice of mandragora, in sub-lethal doses, can stupefy, and hence render a patient less responsive to procedures which would otherwise be extremely painful, its effects – and hence its popularity – were greatly enhanced by the magical properties attributed to it, which made the patient specially susceptible to suggestion. The mandragora or mandrake plant has a bifurcated root, and is supposed in legend to be a sort of living homunculus, half plant and half man. Legendary beliefs about the mandrake are common to many cultures. It is supposed to shriek when pulled from the ground, and anyone who hears the shriek will die. Gatherers of mandrake were therefore supposed to employ a dog, attaching it to the plant by a cord. The struggles of the dog trying to escape would eventually uproot the plant, and the beast would die from hearing the fatal shriek.

Once a plant such as the mandrake has acquired its reputation, it will be used with some efficacy both as a drug and a charm. An Egyptian tablet of 3000 BC refers to it as 'the phallus of the field', and, perhaps following this path, the Babylonians of 2000 BC used a figure cut from the mandrake root as a charm against sterility. A similar belief about the fertility-giving power of the mandrake is shown in the story of Leah and the mandrakes gathered by her son Reuben (Genesis 30: 14–16). Theophrastus, writing as a botanist in the fourth century BC, attributes to mandragora both narcotic and aphrodisiac properties. The Greeks, following the legend of the witch Circe, gave mandragora the name of 'circeum', and its reputation was unabated throughout the succeeding centuries of antiquity. The juice of the white seed of the mandrake plant was known as morion, and Pliny the Elder (AD 24–79) refers to it in the following terms:

> A drachm of it, taken in a draught, or in a cake or other food, causes infatuation, and takes away the use of reason; the person sleeps without sense, in the attitude in which he ate it for three or four hours afterwards. Physicians use it when they have resort to cutting or burning.[5]

(Sir Benjamin Ward Richardson, a nineteenth-century anaesthetist, experimented on himself by drinking a draught containing mandragora, prepared according to a recipe of the ancient Greek surgeon Dioscorides. He described the effects thus:

> The phenomena repeated themselves with all faithfulness, and there can be no doubt that, in the absence of our now more convenient anaesthetics, 'morion' might still be used with some measure of efficacy for general anaesthesia.[6]

Richardson's conclusion is, however, very doubtful. He knew what to expect, and having faith enough to swallow such a draught, no doubt experienced what he expected. Those who do not have such expectancy or faith might not be similarly affected.)

Mandragora's reputation as an anaesthetic lasted until at least the end of the sixteenth century. In The Jew of Malta (c. 1590), Marlowe attributes to it (and to opium) the property of bringing about an absolute and death-like insensibility. 'I drank of poppy and cold mandrake juice,' says Barabas,

> And being asleep, belike they thought me dead,
> And threw me oe'r the walls.[7]

The Traditions of Hippocrates and Asclepius

Greek medicine had two quite distinct traditions running in parallel.

The medicine of the Hippocratic school, although marred by the habit of the ancients of preferring intellectual speculation and debate to empirical research, aspired to be what we would now call scientific. Those who followed this tradition were natural philosophers and physicians. The other tradition was that of religious ritual and centred on the temples dedicated to the god Asclepius, son of Apollo and pupil of Chiron the Centaur. Those who sought help for pain and sickness at the Temples of Sleep, as they were known, were ministered to by priests.

In practice, the Hippocratic physicians paid very little attention to the problem of pain. The fifty odd treatises of the Hippocratic Corpus deal with a variety of medical problems, but pain is not among them. Very little surgery was practised; the two treatises *Fractures* and *Joints* are the ones most concerned with surgery, but their author seems to take for granted that pain must be accepted by the patient. (The Spartan attitude to pain was not confined to Sparta.) It seems strange that these physicians did not do more to alleviate the pain of surgery, for when pain is intense the patient may die of surgical shock. Phillips refers to the fact that in Hippocrates' *Joints*

> The writer mentions with unconcern cases where parts of the thigh or arm may come away of themselves in this condition (gangrene) and notes how lines of demarcation naturally arise between live and dying parts. He would rather not amputate at a place where the limb is fully alive and sentient, because there is a risk of the patient's collapsing from pain and then suddenly dying.[8]

Of course, as Hippocratic physicians were fully aware, there was also a risk of their patients collapsing and dying if given some decoction of analgesic reputation, and they generally preferred that patients should suffer pain rather than run the risk of dying from poisoning at their hands. Galen, the great authority on Hippocratic medicine, finally came to condemn the use of mandragora and similar pain-killing medicines. According to Robinson, he wrote, 'I abhor more than anybody caroctic drugs.'[9] It seems that those who wanted relief from their pain had to turn to the herbal practitioners of folk-medicine, or to the temple medicine of the cult of Asclepius. The extent to which an individual could benefit from the ministrations of the priests would depend upon his own psychological make-up, for the priests used techniques which we would now class as mesmerism or hypnosis, and which are not equally effective with everyone.

The nature of the practices of the priests of Asclepius is known to us chiefly through the Sufi practices which persist to this day in the more remote parts of the Middle East and central Asia. Ja' Far Hallaji[10] relates how he visited a Sufi clinic in Afghanistan in 1961, and witnessed the practice of a form of mesmerism known as *Chuff*; in this, the practitioner repeatedly makes passes over the patient and blows upon him to induce a trance state. This practice resembles very closely that known as *Jar Phoonk*, observed by Esdaile in India in the nineteenth century.[11]

The Sufi technique of inducing therapeutic trances provides a direct link with the cult of Asclepius in ancient Greece. Indeed, the clinic about which Ja' Far Hallaji writes took place in a temple known as the Temple of Sleep.

When medicine declined with the coming of the Dark Ages in the West, it was preserved in Arab culture. Mohammedan writings record that in AD 620 the Prophet put his son-in-law (afterwards the fourth Caliph) into a trance in order painlessly to remove a fragment of a lance which was embedded in his thigh. But pain was not treated entirely by psychological means in the Islamic world. Ibn Sina (AD 980–1037), the great Persian philosopher and physician known in the Christian world as Avicenna, encompassed Greek philosophy and medicine in his scholarship. In contrast to Galen, he advocated the use of herbal drugs for anaesthesia, and his *Canon of Medicine*,[12] translated into Latin, became a standard medical work in Christian Europe for many centuries.

Other Methods of Treating Pain

As well as the herbal and mineral remedies, many manipulative and physical methods of combating pain were in use in antiquity, particularly for the purpose of immediate surgery for battle casualties. The method of pressing on the carotid arteries in the neck, and thus producing transitory unconsciousness, appears to have been widely used in various countries. (The name 'carotid' is related to the Greek word *karoun*, meaning to stupefy.) A related method of producing temporary insensibility and analgesia is to press on the nerve trunks. Pressure on the nerves in the neck may produce some general insensibility (at the risk of producing heart failure!), and pressure on local nerves in a limb may engender a numbness of the part. Keys relates that the ancient Assyrians and Semites were skilled in this practice.[13] It was revived in the sixteenth century by Vivaldi in Italy,[14] and employed as late as the eighteenth century by James Moore.[15]

The conditions under which the wounded were treated on the battlefield led to a useful discovery. If wounded soldiers were left in a half-frozen condition by inadvertent exposure before they were treated, the surgeons found that sometimes the cold had produced a beneficent numbing so that limbs could be amputated without the usual amount of pain. This led to the practice of deliberately freezing injured parts by packing them with ice prior to an operation. This method was revived by Severino[16] in the seventeenth century, and rediscovered by Baron Larrey,[17] a surgeon in Napoleon's army who had much experience of operating on half-frozen soldiers on the battlefield. The method of refrigeration anaesthesia was again revived in the twentieth century, and has various modern applications.[18]

Another curious method of inhibiting pain was by the insertion of needles made of various materials into the subcutaneous tissue at various specified points on the body, the practice known as acupuncture. It is strange that this practice was almost entirely confined to China, where a whole body of medicine grew up around it. Even today there is a great deal of uncertainty as to how the needling inhibits pain, and about the reliability of all the literature connected with it. Undoubtedly, suggestibility plays a large part in acupuncture, but our very recent discoveries about the nature of pain and the neurological mechanisms involved suggest that this is not an entirely adequate explanation for its efficacy in some cases.[19]

Although Chinese medicine was unique in its use of acupuncture, it embraced a formidable *materia medica* as well. The *Great Herbal* which Li Shih-Chen compiled in the sixteenth century from all the famous herbals of ancient times, ran to fifty-two volumes. Many of its remedies are similar to those in use in other lands, although some are uniquely Chinese.

According to the *Chinese Annals of History*,[20] Pien Ch'iao (*c.*BC 250) is supposed to have performed major operations on patients drugged with wine to which some herb was added, and Hua T'o is reported to have used an effervescent powder which, added to wine, produced complete insensibility in patients prior to surgery. The problem with such reports is that one is unsure what degree of credence to give to them. Some are plainly mythical, others may even be intended to be satirical, like the following account attributed to Pien Ch'iao:

> Two men by the name of Lu and Chao visited me. I gave them a subtle drink which reduced them to unconsciousness for three whole days. Then I operated on them and explored the regions of the stomach and heart. I then cut out both stomach and heart and exchanged them in these two persons. Such was the wonderful drug that they uttered no sound, and in a few days I suffered them to return home fully recovered.[21]

As in Hippocratic medicine, surgery was not widely practised in Chinese medicine because of religious prohibitions against mutilating either the living or the dead body. But mythical or not, these accounts of drug-induced anaesthesia for operations show that the problem of pain was considered seriously by the ancient Chinese, and that their extensive interest in herbal medicine extended to attempts at the alleviation of pain when surgery was practised.

In various ancient texts we read accounts of sleep and anaesthesia being induced by getting the patient to inhale vapours. Ingestion of a drug by inhalation rather than by swallowing has the advantage that as soon as unconsciousness is produced, the intoxicant can be withdrawn, whereas once a drug has been swallowed its potency will last for many hours, perhaps with fatal results. Pandit Ballala describes how King Bhoja of Dhar in India, when suffering from severe head pain, was visited by two physicians who decided that they must perform the operation of trepanning the skull. They rendered him unconscious with the fumes of *sammonhini* (probably burning Indian hemp) and after the operation returned him to full consciousness by the administration of another drug called *sanjivini*, the nature of which defies speculation.[22]

The ideal of the effective vapour anaesthetic, which was not realized in practice until the mid nineteenth century, repeatedly occurs in ancient and medieval treatises. It was revived by Hugh of Lucca, a Tuscan physician of the fifteenth century; his son Theodoric describes his father's *oleum de lateribus* as 'a most powerful caustic, and a soporific which, by means of smelling alone, could put patients to sleep on occasion of painful operations which they were to suffer'.

This preparation, which was administered on a sponge, was made up as follows:

> Take of opium, of the juice of the unripe mulberry, of hyoscyamus, of the juice of hemlock, of the juice of the leaves of mandragora, of the juice of the woody ivy, of the juice of the forest mulberry, of the seeds of lettuce, of the seeds of dock, which has large round apples, and of the water hemlock, each an ounce: mix all these in a brazen vessel, and then place in it a new sponge; let the whole boil as long as the sun lasts on the dog-days, until the sponge consumes it all and has boiled away in it. . . . As oft as there shall be need of it, place this sponge in hot water for an hour, and let it be applied to the nostrils of him who is to be operated on until he has fallen asleep, and so let the surgery be performed.[23]

According to some writers, the sleep produced was so profound that the patient would be unconscious for as long as three days, and it would be necessary to awaken him by putting another sponge soaked in vinegar to his nostrils. There is, however, little doubt that the various accounts of the use of the 'sleeping sponge' are largely based upon fantasy and wishful thinking. One can indeed render a person unconscious by stifling him with a wet sponge, but the action is caused by depriving him of air, and if the air supply is withheld for too long, he will surely die. The vapour coming from the various plant-juices may smell pungent but it has little power to enter into the bloodstream and produce unconsciousness or analgesia. Again we have an example of a ritualized practice which can act as a powerful placebo on people who are suitably disposed, and thus help them to bear pain better, for reasons which will be discussed later in this book.

The Acceptance of Pain in Christendom

The early romances convey the impression that sleep-bringing drugs were totally efficacious in producing anaesthesia, and that they were widely used by surgeons for this purpose in Renaissance and pre-Renaissance times. This is totally erroneous. Surgeons could do little more than amputate parts which would otherwise become gangrenous, and apply themselves to patching up wounds. They could not attempt operations which involved opening the abdomen or the chest cavity, because of the inevitable effects of sepsis. Cutting for stones in the bladder was perhaps the most skilful operation attempted. Little attempt was made to mitigate the pain of surgery in Western Europe and in America right up until the mid nineteenth century; instead, patients were often strapped down, or restrained by powerful assistants, so that their struggles did not interfere with the work of the surgeon. As recently as the 1840s, surgeons were still using the barbarous methods of the Middle Ages with rather less concern for the pain of their patients than was shown in the ancient civilizations of Greece and Rome.

The reason for this calm acceptance of pain as the inevitable concomitant of disease, injury and its remedies, has something to do with the attitude of the Christian Church. It was not simply the danger of using herbal remedies such as mandragora, opium and hemp that prevented their general use in practice. It was acknowledged that surgery was also dangerous to life, patients frequently dying from the surgical shock, or later from the subsequent sepsis. Even when ether was discovered and tested on animals to demonstrate its harmlessness, its discoverer, Paracelsus, dared not use it on human beings for fear of offending the Church.

Paracelsus (1490–1541), the name by which Theophrastus Bombastus von Hohenheim chose to call himself, is associated with the early beginnings of a breakaway from traditional medicine and its domination by theology. The Church had enshrined the teachings of Galen and Avicenna - somewhat paradoxically as they were non-Christian - and sought to make all teaching on the subject of man's sickness in relation to his soul's salvation, static. There are many biblical texts that can be interpreted to mean that pain is divinely ordained as a punishment for original sin, and in fact the etymological root of 'pain' is connected with 'penalty'. Attempts to alleviate pain were viewed with grave suspicion by the Church until comparatively modern times. Paracelsus aimed to break with tradition, and he is said to have begun some of his lectures at the University of Basel with a ceremonial burning of works by Galen and Avicenna to symbolize this. He was both a physician and alchemist, and his researches led him to discover the properties of sulphuric ether, the substance which was later to be used widely as an anaesthetic.

Paracelsus distilled alcohol with sulphuric acid and obtained a liquid which he referred to as a 'sulphur', and named it 'sweet vitriol'. He wrote:

> The following should be noted here with regard to this sulphur, that of all things extracted from vitriol it is most remarkable because it is stable. And besides it has associated with it such a sweetness that it is taken even by chickens, and they fall asleep from it for a while but awaken later without harm. On this sulphur no other judgement should be passed than that in diseases which need to be treated with anodynes it quiets all suffering without any harm, and relieves all pain, and quenches all fevers, and prevents complications in all illnesses.[24]

Although this 'sweet vitriol' could have been used safely to permit painless surgery, such a practical step was beyond the daring even of the innovative Paracelsus. Valerius Cordus inherited some of the manuscripts of Paracelsus, and described the properties of the spirit further, recommending it for the treatment of whooping cough. Various later alchemists and chemists re-discovered it, and it was given the name of *spiritus aetherus* in 1730 by Frobenius. It was generally considered to be a compound of sulphuric acid, since that acid was used in its manufacture, and hence regarded with unjustified suspicion as a potent poison.

Paracelsus' discoveries show that we cannot truly attribute the neglect of research into adequate anaesthetics and pain-killers to the lack of sophistication in chemistry and pharmacy which existed right up to the nineteenth century. Unquestionably some part of this neglect must be attributed to an attitude of mind which accepted pain as a simple fact of life. Even in the seventeenth century, when the Church had lost the power to intimidate researchers (who might be accused of witchcraft), physicians failed to interest themselves in the alleviation of pain because the spirit of the times was, by present-day standards, callous and brutal. The infliction of pain out of wanton sport was common. Such sports as bull and bear baiting, cock fighting and dog fighting were taken for granted. Cruel punishments like flogging, and the inhumane execution of offenders, drew interested crowds of spectators seeking thrills. The pain associated with accidents, illnesses and surgery was regarded with a surprising degree of indifference. Even John Evelyn, who appeared to be more civilized and humane than most of his contemporaries in the seventeenth century, regarded witnessing torture as a permissible form of entertainment. On viewing the sights of Paris in 1658, and describing his recreations, he wrote:

> I went to the Chatelet or Prison, where a Malefactor was to have the question or torture given to him, he refusing to confess the robbery with which he was charged: which was thus . . .

Then follows a graphic description of the man first being stretched on the rack, and then being tortured by inflation with water. When the prisoner was 'now to all appearance dead with paine' they finished with him, having got no confession of the robbery he was charged with committing.

Evelyn appears to have had greater sensibility than the other spectators at the show, for he goes on to record:

> There was another Malefactor to succeed, but the spectacle was so uncomfortable, that I was not able to stay the sight of another. It represented yet to me, the intollerable sufferings which our Blessed Saviour must needes undergo when his body was hanging with all its wait upon the nailes on the crosse.[25]

In a society accepting pain, deliberately inflicted or accidental, as a commonplace, it is understandable that little real effort was made to mitigate the pain incidental to disease and its treatment. There were some exceptional individuals such as Ambroise Paré, surgeon to Henry II of France and his three successors, who have gone down in history as renowned humanitarians, and who campaigned against the brutal practices of their colleagues, but a study of the accepted conditions they fought against makes uncomfortable reading.[26]

Much of the foregoing discussion has centred round the pain caused by surgery, for in this matter the doctor knows in advance that painful procedures are going to be undertaken, and can, if he wishes, consider what steps may be taken to avoid the infliction of suffering. But surgery is not the only cause of pain with which medical men have been familiar. Innumerable pathological conditions give great pain, sometimes lasting for years – cancers, kidney stones, arthritis, heart disease and a great range of degenerative diseases. A special kind of pain accompanies, all too often, the coming of each one of us into the world, the pain of childbirth. No other sort of pain exemplifies so strikingly the totally superstitious opposition to giving relief from pain as that endured by women during labour.

Until comparatively recently, women have suffered unnecessarily in giving birth because of a curious male attitude that they ought to suffer in labour. This superstition has found support in the biblical text 'Unto the woman He said, I will greatly multiply thy sorrow and thy conception: in sorrow shalt thou bring forth children' (Genesis 3:16). Midwives have always had some remedies against labour pains, but until recently they have not been too ready to use them because of the prevailing prejudices against rendering such assistance. To provide relief from the pain of childbirth was contrary to the teachings of the Church, and to do so was to run the risk of being accused of witchcraft. It is recorded that Eufame MacAlyne sought the assistance of Agnes Simpson for the relief of labour pains, and for giving such assistance the latter was burnt alive on Castle Hill in Edinburgh in 1591.[27] Yet even after the Chuch had lost its directly coercive power, and when anaesthetics had come into use in surgery in the 1840s, there were priests and religious doctors who still objected strongly to the privilege of relief from pain being extended to women in childbirth. This whole matter will be explored further later in this book, but it is mentioned here to emphasize the point that the search for relief from pain in history has not been hampered solely by inadequate technology and lack of understanding of the mechanisms of pain. Many feminists will regard the long-continued denial of analgesic relief to women in labour as part of the cruel domination of women by men in our history, but while sex-specific attitudes have undoubtedly contributed to it, it is part of a wider bias which some will regard as mere narrow superstition whilst others regard it as an aspect of the religious attitude to life.

The Modern Inheritance

Viewing the whole problem of pain from the perspective of the 1980s, we can see that what has happened is that the problems of acute, transient pain have largely been overcome by technical innovations. We generally consider it wrong that people should be subjected to pain in a dentist's or doctor's surgery. We expect professional therapists to take efficient steps to avoid such an infliction, and by and large they do. But although the problems of acute pain have largely been conquered, the problems of chronic pain have not. According to Devine and Merskey,[28] two out of three patients seeking medical help are complaining of pain. Some of it is acute pain, the useful diagnostic sign of conditions which need attention, but much of it is chronic pain about which the doctor can do very little other than handing out analgesics, tranquillizers, neutral placebos and sympathy. It is little wonder that some experienced and weary physicians come to the conclusion that chronic pain, like the poor, 'will always be with us'. In this they express a view that is basically theological and is bound up with the religious view of guilt and punishment, as discussed by Szasz.[29]

In our modern age, which is characterized by many as irreligious, philosophical conceptualizations alternative to those of the great world religions have had their influence on contemporary thinking. Among them is the outlook associated with the name of Freud, although 'psychoanalytic' has become a convenient shorthand rather than a precisely descriptive term. Freud himself was a confused though influential thinker, and his ideas have been subjected to much damaging criticism by philosophers such as Popper.[30] Implicit in psychoanalytic thinking is the idea that the sufferer may 'need' his symptoms, hence the victim of longstanding pain is in some sense generating it, clinging to it and almost 'enjoying' it. Szasz sees him as *homo dolorosus*, a person who has 'decided' to make a career of pain. Szasz, a somewhat idiosyncratic psychoanalyst, has described the problem of the modern physician dealing with pain patients, in the following terms:

[A] pain situation in which the usual medical approach fails is exemplified by the severely depressed and agitated person who complains of annoying bodily feelings, such as itching, headaches, lack of appetite, insomnia, backache and so forth. Such a person has adopted – fully or partly, permanently or temporarily – the career of being sick and in pain. He does not want his pains allayed or relieved. What is the physician's task in the situation? *Whose* pain should he control: The patient's? That of his relatives, tortured by the patient's complaints? Or his own, generated by his inability to help the patient?[31]

The concept of the doctor taking action appropriate to reducing *his own* pain, is not really fanciful. It is part of the psychoanalytic ploy pithily expressed by the motto, 'If you can't cure the patient – blame him!' Later in this book, in the chapter discussing chronic pain, details will be given of the treatment of chronic pain patients at the Veterans Administration Hospital, San Diego. There, if they fail to secure any improvement in a patient's condition of pain, the doctors may award him a satirical certificate stating that he is a 'Perpetual Pain Patient, who has defeated the best efforts of our specialists, and is to be congratulated on this achievement'.[32]

This reaction to their own failure on the part of a hospital staff represents an interesting backlash against the contemporary belief that doctors *ought* to be able to cure pain, and that they reveal their incompetence if they fail. It may be contrasted with the two arguments which were offered a century ago: first, the theological argument that man had no right to expect to be delivered from pain, because pain was divinely ordained as a punishment for original sin.[33] Second, the brazenly pseudo-scientific argument offered by those surgeons who stoutly maintained that the experience of pain was beneficial for the patient, and it would even aid the healing process.[34] Such arguments are not heard today, and the medical profession must have recourse to alternative ploys in countering the implied criticism that they are often incompetent to deal with chronic pain. These arguments will be pursued further in Chapter 6.

Merskey and Spear,[35] in their discussion of historical attitudes to pain, call attention to the fact that in the nineteenth century, before the introduction of anaesthesia, there was a proper recognition of pain being an experience generated by interaction between both psychological and organic phenomena. They quote Brodie (1837) to the effect that pain in the knee could be hysterical and not due to any direct pathology; in fact Brodie estimated that in 'upper class women' four-fifths of joint pains were hysterical in origin. The term 'hysterical' has come to be such an emotionally loaded word that few of us will frankly admit, 'Yes, I suffer a lot from back pains and they interfere with my work; but there's nothing much wrong with my back – the pains are hysterical'.

Merskey and Spear make the point that the enlightened view of the essential nature of pain which was current in the first half of the nineteenth century became obscured later on by findings in neuro-anatomy and neurophysiology, which generated confidently expressed theories about pain that were mechanistic in nature. It is probable that the zeitgeist of the age, with its rapid development of electrical technology, affected both theories and attitudes to pain. Either the pain was 'really' there (i.e. present as neural impulses travelling up to the brain in postulated 'pain nerves') or it was not. If one tested an electrical circuit one could definitely determine whether or not electrical currents were flowing, so why could not the human body be regarded as a similar piece of apparatus? And if careful examination of the part of a body which the patient claimed to be painful revealed that there was nothing organically wrong, then the pain did not exist and the patient was merely imagining it. Hence arose the accepted convention of classifying pains as either 'organic' or 'psychogenic', a distinction which will be critically discussed throughout this book.

The mechanistic view of pain, which derived from the great scientific and technological advances, and which obscured earlier psychological insights, had gained currency before Freud started writing. The fact that Freud made the impact he did is due to a number of factors, but nowadays he is often credited with an originality that is not wholly justified. Many, if not most, educated people believe that it was Freud who originated ideas such as unconscious motivation, the role of suppressed sexual urges in generating neurotic conflicts and pain, and the mechanisms of hysteria. Almost any historical account of the development of psychological medicine in the nineteenth century reveals that this is very far from the truth.[36] Freud's reputation for originality rests partly on his manner of writing without giving credit to those from whom he took his ideas, and partly because his ideas stood in sharp contrast to the mechanistic ideas that were current in the nineteenth century. The hundred years that followed the great pioneers of neurophysiology and experimental science such as Johannes Müller, Max von Frey and Ernst Weber saw rapid and significant changes in medicine, but it is only comparatively recently that we have been able to tackle the problems of pain which have not been soluble in the existing mechanistic paradigms.

As remarked earlier, the 'psychoanalytic' viewpoint associated with the name of Freud has become a convenient shorthand for an alternative psychological view of pain mechanisms which takes full account of their motivational and affective components. But still later theorists such as Skinner,[37] with his theory of operant conditioning, have added new dimensions to the study and treatment of pain. One does not have to accept the psychoanalytic view, so forcefully put by Szasz, that the chronic sufferer 'needs' his pain. In Skinner's terms, pain may be something which is learnt by operant conditioning – and hence may be unlearnt. The behaviour therapy movement which has burgeoned over the last twenty-five years has provided a theoretical background and a technology whereby pain can be conceptualized and treated in a manner which had not been envisaged prior to the 1950s.

One can hardly mention the advent of the important contribution of psychology to the study and treatment of pain without making special mention of Ronald Melzack, whose fruitful collaboration with Patrick Wall and other neurophysiologists has quite revolutionized the scene.

We now have World Congresses of the International Association for the Study of Pain (the third was in September 1981) which epitomize the concept of interdisciplinary collaboration. Can it be that pain, that ancient enemy, energizer and mocker of mankind, is about to be conquered? In the legend, Prometheus stole fire from heaven and thereby challenged Zeus, who in retaliation let loose upon man the pain and sickness contained in Pandora's box, and chained Prometheus to a rock where he daily endured the torment of an eagle devouring his liver. The latter part of the legend, which is less well known, relates how Hercules slew the eagle and unbound Prometheus, with the consent of Zeus. What the state of man would be after the conquest of pain is difficult to imagine. This book explores what we know of the subject.

REFERENCES

1 Homer, *Iliad*, Book XI, (Trans. Edward Earl of Derby), London: John Murray, 1864, pp. 377-8.

2 See 'Awareness in general anaesthesia', *British Medical Journal*, 22 March, 1980, p. 811.

3 M. Kleiman, 'Histoire de l'anesthésie', *Anesthésie et Analgésie*, 1939, 5, pp. 122-38.

4 See Matthew 27:34; Mark 15:23 and 36; Luke 23:36; John 19:29.

5 Pliny the Elder, quoted in *Anaesthetics Antient and Modern*, London: Burroughs, Wellcome & Co., 1907, p. 19.

6 B. W. Richardson, *Disciples of Aesculapius*, London: Hutchinson, 1900, p. 147.

7 I. Ribner (ed.), *The Complete Plays of Christopher Marlowe*, New York: Odyssey, 1963.

8 Cited by E. D. Phillips, *Greek Medicine*, London: Thames & Hudson, 1973, p. 103.

9 Galen, cited by V. Robinson, *Victory Over Pain: A History of Anaesthesia*, London: Sigma Books, 1947, p. 21.

10 Ja' Far Hallaji, 'Hypnotherapeutic techniques in a Central Asian community', *International Journal of Clinical and Experimental Hypnosis*, 1962, 10, pp. 271-4.

11 See J. Esdaile, *Mesmerism in India and Its Practical Application in Surgery and Medicine*, London: Longman, Brown, Green & Longmans, 1846.

12 See G. Sarton, *Introduction to the History of Science*, Vol. 1, Baltimore: Carnegie Institute, 1927.

13 T. E. Keys, *The History of Surgical Anaesthesia*, New York: Dover Publications, 1963.

14 Cited by M. Kleiman, 'Histoire de l'anesthésie', opt. cit.

15 J. Moore, *A Method of Preventing or Diminishing Pain in Several Operations of Surgery*, London: T. Cadell, 1784.

16 M. A. Severino, 'Use of snow and ice for surgical anaesthesia', cited in F. H. Garrison, *An Introduction to the History of Medicine*, 4th Edition, Philadelphia: W. B. Saunders & Co., 1929, p. 824.

17 D. J. Larrey, 'No pain in amputations at very low temperatures' (1807), in J. T. Gwathmey (ed.), *Anaesthesia*, 2nd Edition, New York: Macmillan, 1924.

18 See J. W. Lloyd, 'Experiences in a pain relief unit, 1970–1976', in A. W. Harcus, R. Smith and B. Whittle (eds), *Pain: New Perspectives in Management*, London: Churchill Livingstone, 1977.

19 See F. B. Mann, *The Treatment of Disease by Acupuncture*, London: Heinemann, 1974.

20 See K. C. Wong and Wu Lien-Teh, *History of Chinese Medicine*, Shanghai: National Quarantine Service, 1936.

21 Cited by G. Bankoff, *The Conquest of Pain*, London: Macdonald & Co., 1955, p. 18.

22 See G. Mukhopadhyaya, *History of Indian Medicine*, Calcutta: University of Calcutta, 1923.

23 Cited by T. E. Keys, *The History of Surgical Anaesthesia*, op. cit.

24 Cited by V. Robinson, *Victory Over Pain*, op. cit., p. 35.

25 J. Evelyn, *Memoirs*, (ed. William Bray), London: A. Murray & Son, 1871, p. 210.

26 See F. R. Packard, *Life and Times of Ambroise Paré*, London: Oxford University Press, 1922.

27 See H. W. Haggard, *Devils, Drugs and Doctors*, New York: Harper & Bros, 1929.

28 R. Devine and H. Merskey, 'The description of pain in psychiatric and general medical patients', *Journal of Psychosomatic Research*, 1965, 9, pp. 311–16.

29 T. Szasz, *Pain and Pleasure*, New York: Basic Books, 1957.

30 K. R. Popper, *Conjectures and Refutations*, London: Routledge & Kegan Paul, 1963.

31 T. Szasz, 'A psychiatric perspective on pain and its control', in F. D. Hart (ed.), *The Treatment of Chronic Pain*, Lancaster: Medical and Technical Books, 1974, p. 43.

32 See R. A. Sternbach, *Pain Patients: Traits and Treatments*, New York: Academic Press, 1974, p. 107.

33 For an account of the theological argument against the relief of pain, see H. W. Haggard, *Devils, Drugs and Doctors*, op. cit.

34 For reference to the argument that pain was beneficial and healing in surgery, see J. Elliotson, *Numerous Cases of Surgical Operations Without Pain in the Mesmeric State*, London: H. Baillière, 1843.

35 H. Merskey and F. G. Spear, *Pain: Psychological and Psychiatric Aspects*, London: Baillière Tindall & Cassell, 1967.

36 For different but complementary accounts of the development of dynamic psychiatry in the nineteenth century see H. F. Ellenberger, *The Discovery of the Unconscious*, London: Allen Lane, 1970, and M. D. Altschule, *Roots of Modern Psychiatry*, New York: Grune & Stratton, 1965.

37 B. F. Skinner, *Science and Human Behavior*, New York: Macmillan, 1953.

2

THE BEGINNINGS OF MODERN ANAESTHESIA

Joseph Priestley and Humphrey Davy

In the previous chapter it was related how sporadic efforts had been made throughout history to bring about unconsciousness by means of inhaling vapours. Although never very effective in ancient medicine, this practice was also never very dangerous because some such device as the 'sleeping sponge' could always be withdrawn when the patient showed signs of being deeply unconscious, and he would then revive by inhaling pure air. In the late eighteenth century there was renewed interest in inhalants as anaesthetics, led by the work of Joseph Priestley.

Priestley, a dissenting minister, was a polymath who directed his energies and interests into many fields. He was awarded the degree of Doctor of Laws by Edinburgh University for a thesis on education, but it was his meeting with Benjamin Franklin in London which first turned his interests to science. He was admitted to the Royal Society at the age of thirty-three on the strength of his *History of Electricity*, a subject dear to Franklin's heart. Whilst pastor of a chapel in Leeds, Priestley chanced to live next to a brewery, and there he became fascinated with the phenomenon of 'fixed air', as carbon dioxide was then called, which lay like a gaseous blanket over the vats. He became a self-taught chemist, and was awarded the Copley Medal by the Royal Society for his work on gases.[1]

Priestley's chief claim to fame lies in his discovery of oxygen. He seems to have regarded it as some sort of basic elixir of life, and suggested that it might become 'an article of luxury' which the rich could inhale for their health and pleasure. However, it was the French chemist Lavoisier, with whom Priestley corresponded, who realized the true importance of oxygen in chemistry, and how an understanding of its properties demolished the ancient phlogiston theory.

Priestley devoted much effort to the isolation and collection of various gases. This work integrated well with the development of a new school of medicine, Dr Beddoes' 'Pneumatic Medicine'. Beddoes proceeded on the principle that hithertofore drugs had been administered by the mouth to be ingested by the stomach and intestines, often with dire results when the dose did not suit the constitution of the patient. By administering drugs by inhalation into the lungs a far greater control of dosage, and of monitoring by outcome, could be achieved. The various new gases which Priestley was isolating were thus employed in the Pneumatic Institute at Clifton. Not only was oxygen employed, but nitrogen and hydrogen too, as therapy for diseases such as consumption and asthma. The movement for Pneumatic Medicine soon progressed to a point where a wide variety of diseases were being treated, without any clear rationale, by whatever gases took the doctors' fancy.

Among the gases prepared by Priestley was nitrous oxide, later to be known as 'laughing gas' because of its property of inducing exhilaration when inhaled in small quantities. But Priestley's gas was very impure and therefore poisonous when inhaled in any quantity. Although Priestley discovered this gas in 1772, it remained a scientific curiosity until 1795 when Humphrey Davy prepared a purer form of it and experimented with it upon himself. Davy was at that time a precocious youth of seventeen, working as an assistant to a Dr Borlase, and he noted that inhalation of the gas produced a sense of giddiness and exhilaration, with a general feeling of exaltation.

In 1798, at the age of twenty-one, Davy was appointed chemical superintendent of Beddoes' Pneumatic Institute, and given facilities to pursue researches into the properties of the various gases in use. In 1800 he published an important treatise entitled *Researches, Chemical and Philosophical, Chiefly Concerning Nitrous Oxide or Dephlogisticated Nitrous Air and its Respiration*. In this treatise he gave details of his experiments on himself, including the following passages:

> In cutting one of the unlucky teeth called dentes sapientiae, I experienced an extensive inflammation of the gum, accompanied with great pain, which equally destroyed the power of response and of consistent action.
>
> On the day when the inflammation was most troublesome, I breathed three large doses of nitrous oxide. The pain always diminished after the first four or five respirations; the thrilling came as usual, and uneasiness was for a few minutes swallowed up in pleasure. As the former state of mind returned, the state of the organ returned with it; and I once imagined that the pain was more severe after the experiment than before. . . .
>
> As nitrous oxide in its extensive operation appears capable of destroying physical pain, it may probably be used with advantage

during surgical operations in which no great effusion of blood takes place.[2]

Here we have a publication by a reputable chemist, shortly afterwards to be elected a fellow of the Royal Society, which plainly pointed the way to effective and safe analgesia in surgery. Yet because of an astonishingly ingrained conservativism among the medical fraternity humanity had to wait another forty-six years before effective efforts were made to alleviate the pain of surgical operations – and then, not by the initiative of a medical man but by a dentist.

Davy was a true scientist in that he realized the psychological as well as the pharmacological effect of breathing gases alleged to be anaesthetic in action. After describing the effects of a mixture of nitrous oxide and air on a young woman who had been the subject of 'hysteric fits' and was therefore not to be trusted in her subjective report of the effect of the gas, he then performed a further control experiment on another young woman who was not given to hysteric imaginings. First, in order to 'ascertain the influence of imagination', he gave her a bag of 'common air', which she declared 'produced no effect'.[3] Only then did he administer a gas-air mixture and note the manifest analgesic and behavioural effects of its chemical properties.

Davy's experiments with nitrous oxide aroused interest among his colleagues and friends. He prepared gas-bags made of close-woven silk material, and got his friends to try the gas. Samuel Taylor Coleridge, who was always interested in drugs and strange experiences, reported thus:

> The first time I inspired the nitrous oxide I felt an highly pleasurable sensation of warmth over my whole frame, resembling that which I remember once to have experienced after returning from a walk in the snow into a warm room. The only motion which I felt inclined to make, was that of laughing at those who were looking at me. . . . The third time I was more violently acted on than in the two former. Towards the last, I could not avoid, nor indeed felt any wish to avoid, beating the ground with my feet: and after the mouthpiece was removed, I remained in a few seconds in great extacy.[4]

Betty McQuitty quotes Coleridge writing elsewhere of his experiences under nitrous oxide:

> I experienced the most voluptious sensations. The outer world grew dim, and I had the most entrancing visions. For three and a half minutes I lived in a world of new sensations.[5]

(Coleridge, of course, had a powerful imagination, which undoubtedly contributed to his psychological experiences when under the influence of nitrous oxide. Those of us who are blessed with less creative imaginations cannot expect to obtain such ecstatic experiences from the gas.)

Coleridge might have become addicted to gas-sniffing, as he was to opium, for he suffered continuously from various pains. Drug-use, at the end of the eighteenth century and the beginning of the nineteenth, was almost epidemic in its proportions. Opium was used by all classes of the population, not simply as a pain-killer but as a substitute for alcohol, for during this period the desired effects could be achieved more cheaply with opium pills than with gin or other liquor.

As nitrous oxide was a comparative rarity and under the control of research chemists, it did not become a common article of commerce like opium. However, in the hospital laboratories and other places where men of science and their students gathered, the gas was frequently used out of interest, and indeed for entertainment. Allen, a chemistry lecturer at Guy's Hospital, recorded the following in 1800:

> Present, Astley Cooper, Bradley Fox and others. We all breathed the gaseous oxide of azote [nitrous oxide]. It took a surprising effect on me, abolishing at first all sensations; then I had the idea of being carried violently upward in a dark cavern with only a few glimmering lights. The company said that my eyes were fixed, face purple, veins in the head very large, apoplectic stertor. They were all much alarmed, but I suffered no pain and in a short time came to myself.[6]

As will be described later, sniffing nitrous oxide for fun, and for the entertainment it provided to spectators, became a fairground act in the United States in the early part of the nineteenth century, and it was out of this showman's business that it came to the serious attention of a dentist who finally put it to good use in the painless extraction of teeth.

Although the early promise of Beddoes' Pneumatic Medicine was not fulfilled, gases continued to be used for therapeutic if not for anaesthetic purposes at the beginning of the nineteenth century. Dr J. C. Warren, who was later to play an important role in the introduction of ether as an anaesthetic for surgery, used the vapour as early as 1805 to relieve inflammation of the lungs; it never occurred to him that such vapour could induce a beneficent unconsciousness if given in sufficient quantity.[7] Michael Faraday noted that, 'When the vapour of ether mixed with common air is inhaled, it produced effects very similar to those occasioned by nitrous oxide,'[8] but he, like other scientists, did not apply this discovery to the alleviation of clinical pain.

It is not entirely true that doctors neglected to apply the scientific knowledge of their time to the conquest of pain. There were exceptional individuals who tried to do this. What is remarkable is the cold reception such pioneers received from their orthodox medical colleagues when they tried to promote new, humane techniques. It was almost as if the medical fraternity, no longer oppressed by religious superstitions concerning pain, were still maintaining these attitudes out of sheer conservatism. Medical historians are apt to gloss over the very questionable record of their profession in opposing humane innovations in this period of the early nineteenth century, but the fact is that their opposition was finally overcome by the efforts of quacks, mesmerists and dentists.

Henry Hickman

As an example of the shabby treatment accorded to a medical man who stepped out of line in trying to bring the benefits of anaesthesia to medical practice, we may quote the case of Henry Hickman (1800–1830). Hickman was an extremely bright young man, who became a member of the London Royal College of Surgeons at the age of twenty, and was admitted to the Royal Medical Society of Edinburgh soon after. He began his career as a general practitioner in Ludlow, Shropshire. According to the author of an article in the *British Medical Journal* which sought to rehabilitate his name after a century of neglect, Hickman was 'impressed by the agonizing sufferings of those on whom he was called to operate', and he 'resolved to seek some method of alleviating their pain by rendering them unconscious before the operation.'

With this object he commenced a series of experiments on animals, first by producing semi-asphyxiation by the exclusion of atmospheric air; then by causing them to inhale small quantities of carbon dioxide, and later nitrous oxide gas. After rendering the animals unconscious, he excised the ears, amputated their legs, made incisions, then dressed the wounds, then noted the time they took to heal, and the period of their complete recovery. He carried on these experiments for some time and at last met with considerable success. This convinced him that, could he but carry out his experiments on the human subject, his methods would become of the greatest value to mankind in making painless the performance of major surgical operations.[9]

Hickman noted that in his earliest type of experiment where the animal was denied atmospheric air, it 'showed great marks of uneasiness' before it became unconscous; but in the later type of experiment, where it was put directly into an atmosphere of carbon dioxide, it would become unconscious in one minute. Under both conditions surgical operations could be performed whilst the animal was unconscious without it showing any signs of pain. The animals would recover consciousness apparently showing no ill effects other than the surgery which had been performed upon them. (Nowadays one might look for the more subtle signs resulting from cerebral anoxia, particularly in human subjects.)

What Hickman had done was to apply the same principle as in the ancient Assyrian method of pressing on the carotid arteries to produce unconsciousness. The effects of this manipulation are rather complex: first, it cuts off the supply of freshly oxygenated blood to the brain cells; second, it floods the brain with self-generated carbon dioxide. The physiology of cerebral anoxia and raising the level of cellular carbon dioxide is not wholly understood even today. It is a highly dangerous practice in that it may cause irreversible brain damage if continued too long, but the mature brain appears to be remarkably robust (in contrast to the infant brain) in tolerating this phenomenon. Over a century ago, when judicial executions by hanging involved leaving the culprit to asphyxiate in the hangman's noose, it was not unknown for friends of hanged felons to cut down the body from the gallows and revive it.[10]

Hickman experimented with both carbon dioxide and nitrous oxide as inhalants, and satisfied himself that he could perform painless operations successfully. He knew, however, that before he could apply his methods to human beings he would need the backing of influential patrons. His first approach was to T. A. Knight, President of the Royal Horticultural Society, who was an F.R.S., and hence familiar with Humphrey Davy and Michael Faraday. Knowing that both these distinguished scientists had predicted a time when gaseous inhalations would be used to abolish pain in surgical operations, Hickman had high hopes that his innovatory experiments would receive their patronage. In 1824 he produced a pamphlet entitled 'A letter on suspended animation, containing experiments showing that it may safely be employed during operations on animals, with a view to ascertaining its probable utility in surgical operations on the human subject, addressed to T. A. Knight Esq., of Downton Castle, Herefordshire, one of the Presidents of the Royal Society'.

Knight, although an F.R.S., was not a 'President of the Royal Society'; by this gaffe Hickman showed his ignorance, and probably incurred the contempt of Davy, who was now Sir Humphrey Davy, and President of the Royal Society. Davy declined to give his patronage to this obscure young country doctor. One might have expected a more humane response from Michael Faraday, who was less of a social lion, but perhaps he too felt a certain guilt that he had done nothing about his earlier observations on the anaesthetic properties of ether vapour. Both men snubbed Hickman.

The best Hickman could achieve was permission to read a paper to the Medical Society of London, describing his researches with animals and his projects for the future. The paper was poorly received and, disheartened by the attitude of the medical establishment in England, Hickman went to Paris to try his luck with the French *Académie des Sciences*. This body had a reputation for greater enlightenment, and had even taken the claims of the mesmerists sufficiently seriously to appoint repeated commissions of inquiry. Hickman wrote a petition to Charles X of France asking for his claims to be investigated, and Charles referred the matter to a Dr Guérardin, who prepared a report to the *Académie*. This report, presented in October 1828, was greeted by the leading physicians and surgeons with contempt and ridicule. Its sole champion was Baron Larrey, the old army surgeon of Napoleon's *Grande Armée*, who had done much to ease the sufferings of soldiers on the battlefield. Hickman's proposals obviously had their dangers, but the expectancy of death through surgical shock and later sepsis was so great in major operations at that time, that it would at least have been reasonable to have instituted a research programme on gaseous anaesthesia. Hickman returned to England and died soon afterwards at the age of twenty-nine.

The medical establishment has since made something of a martyr of Hickman. In 1930 a memorial to him was unveiled at the church in Bromfield, Shropshire, where he is buried, and there was a memorial gathering at the Wellcome Museum in his honour, addressed by Lord Dawson of Penn.[11] He is now a celebrated figure in British medical history, a hero in the official saga of how the medical profession rescued suffering humanity from pain. When such heroes of the past are canonized they bespeak of a collective guilty conscience, and one wonders how many Henry Hickmans are struggling to get their findings recognized today.

Robert Collyer: Alcohol and Mesmerism

The case of Robert Collyer is another example of the medical profession's strange reluctance to come to grips with the problem of pain. It is not easy to find information about this remarkable man, for his name, spelt variously Collyer and Collier, appears in few biographies. He is not mentioned among the 500 odd pioneers of anaesthesia in Thomas Keys' *History of Surgical Anaesthesia*,[12] or in Gwathmey's *Anaesthesia*,[13] nor yet in Garrison's *Introduction to the History of Medicine*.[14] Lesser medical authorities, if they mention him, tend to dismiss him rather contemptuously, for reasons which will become clear.

Collyer is unique in that he experimented with alcohol as an inhalant in the relief of pain. Since immemorial times alcohol has been used as a specific against pain, but as a drink. As we have seen, many of the ancient drugs like mandragora and hellebore were given in rather conservatively small quantities, but in wine, the latter being the safer pharmacological agent. Sufferers from pain have often turned to alcoholic drinks for relief, and chronic sufferers may become drunkards. Even today the final medical remedy for pain in terminal cancer, when the patient has only a few more months to live, is the so-called 'Brompton cocktail' – gin 1.5 ml, morphine sulphate 15 mg, cocaine 10 mg, water or syrup up to 5 ml.[15] Up to the middle of the nineteenth century wounded sailors and soldiers were often given a very large tot of rum before the surgeon got to work on them, and it is even reported that some surgeons in civil life went to the operating theatre with two bottles of spirits, one for the unfortunate patient and one to sustain the nerve of the operator at his grisly task.

The problem about drinking alcohol to provide anaesthesia is as follows. The alcohol is first absorbed by the lining of the stomach and intestine into the bloodstream, and immediately acts in low concentration by stimulating the rostral end of the reticular formation in the brain, thus livening up the cerebral cortex. But as the concentration of alcohol in the blood rises, it soon begins to act as a cerebral depressant. This term 'depressant' may be confusing to the layman, because the immediate effect is some elevation of mood and euphoria. The parts of the brain which are first depressed are the 'higher' centres; the drinker feels less thoughtful, less anxious and more relaxed. This euphoria has an immediate effect on pain; indeed, according to Ellis,[16] the threshold of pain may be raised by as much as 40 per cent by a few stiff drinks. Not only is alcohol a euphoric in its action on the central nervous system, but its action on the peripheral nervous system is analgesic in a manner similar to aspirin. Some drinkers report that at a certain stage of intoxication they feel the skin of their face, or some other area of the body, go numb.

A consideration of the different levels of alcohol in the blood is instructive with regard to their psychological and physiological effects. With an alcohol concentration of over 0.01 per cent, the individual may be called 'drunk' to the extent that he is not safe to drive a car. Actually, intoxication varies very much with such factors as the health of the individual, and with his type of personality.[17] More extraverted people will become 'drunk' on less alcohol than more introverted people. The higher the level of blood alcohol the more generally disorganized, mentally and physically, the individual becomes, until somewhere around the level of 0.5 per cent he will become unconscious. But this level is dangerously near to the fatal level, for should it rise much above 0.55 per cent he may die, because the alcohol impairs vital functions such as breathing and heartbeat. Ether in the blood is far safer because there is a much wider margin between the concentration producing unconsciousness and that which may be fatal.

If a large quantity of neat spirits is swallowed, a surprising and paradoxical consequence ensues. The lining of the stomach and intestine reacts by becoming irritated and the rate of the absorption of alcohol is slowed up. Wine with a concentration of about 20 per cent alcohol is more immediately intoxicating than neat spirits with a 40 to 50 per cent concentration; thus at functions such as weddings and cocktail parties the drinking of champagne or spirits diluted with fruit juice secures exhilaration and social relaxation more quickly than if neat spirits were being consumed. Taking alcohol by the mouth means that it becomes absorbed into the contents of the stomach and intestines and slowly diffuses into the bloodstream. A dose of swallowed alcohol sufficient to render a man unconscious therefore has to be a very large one indeed. The contents of the gut are drenched in it and the whole system is poisoned for many hours. Although alcohol is excreted in the urine, breath and sweat, this accounts for only a small proportion of it. About 90 per cent of it has to be metabolized by the body, and in the course of this process the person may become very ill.

In view of the above facts it is obvious that the drinking of alcoholic liquors as a means of achieving anaesthesia has many drawbacks and dangers. Robert Collyer's contribution to the whole movement of research into anaesthetics was to recommend not the drinking of alcoholic liquor, but the inhalation of vapourized alcohol. By this method the drug is absorbed immediately into the bloodstream through the lungs and rapidly builds up a concentration sufficient to render the brain unconscious. The supply can then immediately be withdrawn, and the patient is left with no surplus alcohol in his system.

It had been known for a long time that those working in cellars bottling wine might become intoxicated simply by breathing the vapour. Collyer's first experience of encountering anaesthesia induced by alcohol vapour was when he was called to assist a Negro youth who had been rendered unconscious by the fumes in a rum vat on the estate of Collyer's father in New Orleans. The youth had fallen unconscious, and in doing so had dislocated his hip. Collyer found him quite relaxed, and reduced the dislocated joint without causing him any pain; the boy awoke later having suffered no ill effects from the accident or the anaesthesia.

Collyer had studied medicine at University College, London, where he was present at a lecture given by Professor Edward Turner, who demonstrated the properties of ether to his students. By sniffing it, Collyer experienced a transient unconsciousness, and he noted that his fellow students became insensible to pain under its influence.

At the same time, 1835, Dr John Elliotson was practising mesmerism at University College Hospital, then known as the North London Hospital, and held out hopes for its general use in the abolition of pain in surgery. The story of Elliotson's struggle to get mesmerism accepted by the medical profession, particularly in relation to its use in overcoming pain in surgery, is well known. Although he was appointed Professor of the Theory and Practice of Medicine in 1831, and was a man of enormous prestige and influence, he was forced to resign in 1839 because of his championship of mesmeric practices.

Collyer, who, like Hickman, was determined to find an answer to the problem of pain in surgery, studied the effects of mesmerism and the inhalation of vapours and came to the conclusion that the anaesthetic state produced by either means was the same. For more than a century this was regarded as a crass error, but in the 1970s research revealed facts which imply that this idea may not be such a misconception, as will be discussed later in this book.

Collyer was judged to be a crank in two respects; he not only questioned the wisdom of his elders with regard to the allegedly outrageous practice of stupefying patients by inhalations before surgery, but he also dabbled in mesmerism. When he later went to America, he performed operations on patients claiming that he had rendered them anaesthetic by mesmeric influence. In some cases he used the vapour of alcohol, preferring it to ether, possibly because it was easier to obtain a vapour of pure ethyl alcohol than of sulphuric ether, as the commercial variety of the latter was often very contaminated. In 1840 he went on a tour of America lecturing on both mesmerism and on anaesthesia produced by inhalation. Such an approach was unlikely to bring Collyer either fame or respectability, as at that time there were many itinerant lecturers and showmen in America, some calling themselves 'Doctor' and 'Professor', many of whom were arrant quacks. Nevertheless, the activities of these men, who were often half-educated and possessed no more than a smattering of medical, dental and scientific knowledge, stirred up a demand among the public that the medical and dental professions should try to do more about the problem of pain. Anyone could set up as a mesmerist, and because the patient's response to mesmerism is more a function of his own natural ability to experience trance phenomena than any special skill of the mesmerist, quacks could often perform minor surgery and dentistry painlessly with patients who knew from bitter experience that an orthodox doctor would have caused them excruciating pain.

In 1843 Collyer returned to Liverpool and continued his lectures and demonstrations of both mesmerism and of narcosis by alcoholic vapour. He had not got a very firm grasp of the principles of anaesthesia, for he macerated poppy heads and coriander in the alcohol he used to produce the vapour, substances which would not increase the effectiveness of the vapour because of their lack of volatility. However, his errors must be regarded in the context of the crass ignorance of much chemistry and physiology by the medical profession of his time. After the 1840s he produced no more interesting work.

A pamphlet published by Burroughs and Wellcome at the turn of the century pays a rare tribute to Collyer. It is one of the few writings on the history of anaesthesia that does not belittle or ignore his contribution. His lectures, it states,

> excited general attention at the time and there is little doubt that they gave a fresh impetus to research on the subject of anaesthesia by inhalation. He must therefore be regarded as an important pioneer, who, had he given up his ideas of mesmerism and proceeded systematically with his plan of making the body insensible by inhaling the vapour of alcohol, would have had no one to dispute with him in priority.[18]

It is perhaps natural that a pamphlet published by a drug firm should be biased to the pharmacological aspects of anaesthesia and imply that Collyer should have 'given up his ideas of mesmerism'; but if Collyer had been a more gifted resarcher, a blending of his two interests might have had more fruitful results in unravelling the mysteries of pain.

Anaesthetic Innovations in Dentistry

If members of the medical profession were discouraged from research into chemical anaesthetics partly by conservatism and partly out of fear of losing their good name, others were not so constrained. Medical students, for instance, were less burdened by the pressures of respectability than their elders, and the first recorded case of the painless extraction of a tooth with the use of ether anaesthesia is that by a student called William Clarke at Berkshire Medical College, USA, in 1842. After experimenting with ether for the purpose of enjoying 'ether frolics' with his friends, Clarke obtained sufficient expertise in the administration of the vapour to give just enough to make the inhaler pass through the initial stage of excitement and become unconscious with safety. He is reported to have anaesthetized a Miss Hobby by giving ether on a towel, so that a dentist, Elijah Pope, could extract a tooth painlessly.[19]

It was a chemist, Gardner Q. Colton, like Collyer a former student of Edward Turner at University College, London, who was largely instrumental in bringing anaesthesia to dentistry and surgery in America. (There were later many other claimants to this honour who had doubtless made independent discoveries on their own account.) Colton, not being a physician, was not constrained by considerations of professional etiquette, and was making a living by travelling around giving 'lectures' on chemistry, which were really no more than entertaining exhibitions of people getting drunk on a little nitrous oxide. His custom was to hire a hall and advertise a lecture, broadly hinting that the performance would be uproariously funny. One poster advertising such an event in 1845 states among other things, 'Probably no one will attempt to fight'.[20]

In December 1844 Gardner Colton organized such a lecture and demonstration in Hartford, Connecticut. Among the audience was a local dentist, Horace Wells. Wells noticed that one of the young men who became excited by the gas banged his shin severely in the course of his antics, but appeared to take no notice of the injury. When Wells later asked him whether he was aware how hard he had hit his leg, the man was quite surprised to find that it was injured, and declared that he had felt no pain. Wells then realized that as well as provoking intoxication, the gas could induce a remarkable degree of analgesia.

Wells then approached Colton, who agreed to come to the dental surgery next day and administer nitrous oxide to Wells himself, who needed to have one of his own teeth extracted. The anaesthesia was successfully accomplished, and a dentist colleague pulled out the tooth without Wells feeling pain, observers testifying that he appeared to be unconscious during the process.

Wells was an impetuous man and wanted immediately to introduce the practice of anaesthetizing his patients when there was painful dentistry to be done. His dental colleague Riggs was more cautious and advised him to seek the advice of a well-known doctor and chemist, Charles Jackson. Another dental colleague, William Morton, was actually staying with Jackson at the time, and he and Wells consulted him together in January 1845. Jackson warned of the dangers of giving nitrous oxide in any quantity because of the possibility that a patient might die under its influence, a danger that was real, and was overcome only many years later when the correct proportions of gas and oxygen for safe administration were established.[21] Wells, however, was not to be dissuaded, and having got Colton to show him how to prepare nitrous oxide, he proceeded to use it in his practice, apparently with some initial success.

Wells' next attempt to seek some authoritative sanction for his anaesthetic practice was to apply to Dr John C. Warren of the Massachusetts General Hospital at Boston. He hoped that Warren, an eminent surgeon, would allow him to administer nitrous oxide to a patient undergoing an amputation, but Warren demurred at taking such a responsibility, and instead permitted Wells to address a gathering of medical students at Harvard Medical School and to demonstrate a dental extraction using the gas. Accounts of what took place vary, but two things seem to have gone wrong. First, neither Wells nor William Morton who was assisting him, was particularly adept at administering the gas and they were too chary of giving an overdose; second, the audience had not been fully briefed so that they would understand that when lightly anaesthetized a patient may nevertheless moan aloud although experiencing no pain. Although, according to Keys,[22] the patient afterwards declared that he had felt no pain, he had moaned aloud during the demonstration. The students jeered at Wells, and the cause of nitrous oxide anaesthesia was not advanced. After some more experimentation with the gas in his private practice, Wells abandoned dentistry altogether. Morton persisted, turning to ether as an alternative agent.

The Success of Ether Anaesthesia

Although not a man of great scientific education, Morton proceeded in a more systematic manner than Wells. He experimented with the effect of ether vapour on various animals, and finally upon himself, suffering no ill effects. He then went on to try the vapour on other humans, prevailing upon two assistants to be subjects of the experiment. The result was highly disturbing, for instead of a period of slight excitement followed by a quiet unconsciousness, both young men became violently intoxicated on inhalation. Trying the vapour again himself, he found that his own response was violent and quite unlike his earlier experience. Clearly something had gone very wrong, and in his puzzlement he once more sought the advice of Dr Charles Jackson.

In taking such a course, Morton was justifiably suspicious that the latter might try to claim credit for what he was trying to accomplish for himself, for Morton fully intended to patent the process of anaesthesia commercially if he were successful with it. Jackson had previously been involved in a long litigation with Morse over who had the real right to claim to be the inventor of the electric telegraph. Morton did not take Jackson into his confidence, but approached him in general terms, discussing the properties of ether. Later he admitted:

> I went to Dr Jackson's therefore to procure a gas-bag, also with the intention of ascertaining something more accurately as to the different preparations of ether, if I should find I could do so without setting him on the track of experiment with myself.[23]

By discreet questioning, Morton managed to find out from Jackson that there were different grades of ether, and that the spirit might even deteriorate over time. Jackson advised him to use only the most highly rectified, and told him where he might purchase it. He also showed him how to use a glass flask with a projecting tube, rather than the gas-bag Morton had asked for, and lent him such an apparatus. On the strength of this advice and help, Jackson was later to feel that Morton had tricked him, and picked his brains by deceit. When Morton eventually became famous, Jackson's paranoid fury was aroused to a great pitch of vindictiveness, and he hotly contested Morton's claim to be the originator of ether anaesthesia.

It was now clear to Morton why his second series of experiments had been so disastrous; the ether in his second stock had been of the impure commercial variety. Benefiting from Jackson's advice about the necessary degree of purity of the liquid, and about an improved method of administering the vapour, he returned to his experiments and found that the rectified spirit was safe to use. Interestingly, the first patient who came to him demanding help was a man in great pain who said he feared to have his tooth drawn, and asked if Morton could produce anaesthesia by *mesmerism*.[24] Morton was well aware of the current practice of mesmerism for the relief of pain, and had joked about it with Jackson, suggesting that an empty gas-bag might be a sufficient 'prop' to induce an analgesic trance in a suitably impressionable subject. However, he told this patient that he had something better than mesmerism to offer him, and anaesthetized him by the very simple method of holding a handkerchief saturated with ether over his face. This man, Eben Frost, was to become a staunch supporter of Morton, and gave him a testimonial, countersigned by the dental assistant Hayden, describing the successful painless operation.

It will be apparent that the whole campaign for the successful launching of ether anaesthesia in America was essentially a *commercial* one. The medical profession had failed, from either a scientific or a humanitarian point of view, to do anything about the problem of pain in surgery. It took the thrust of American capitalist enterprise to inaugurate a revolution that was to spread rapidly throughout the civilized world. This important fact is often overlooked, and it suggests the interesting rider that in our present age prevailing attitudes to, and practices dealing with, problems of pain, are very much conditioned by commercial considerations which stress the *pharmacological* control of pain, rather than conceptualizing the problem in alternative terms.

Morton lost no time in advertising his painless methods of dentistry in the Boston *Daily Journal*, and set out to attract custom. In order to satisfy the public that the methods he was using were harmless, he tried to get a testimonial from Dr Jackson, whose scientific authority was widely respected. Jackson, feeling that he had been exploited, refused to provide one. In fact, he was not entirely sure just what Morton was doing, although he later came to a financial arrangement with Morton when the latter took out a patent on his process of anaesthesia. Jackson suggested, not without some justification, that a man like Morton with such limited scientific and medical knowledge, might well kill a patient he was anaesthetizing.

Much of the credit for the introduction of anaesthesia in surgery must go to John Warren, the famous surgeon who had permitted Wells to try to demonstrate to the Harvard medical students the powers of nitrous oxide. Undeterred by this fiasco, Warren was prepared to listen sympathetically when Morton approached him through the intermediary of a young surgeon, H. J. Bigelow, who had seen Morton's methods and appreciated their possibilities. Morton also had the ear of Mason Warren, the son of the great man, who was studying surgery. Morton's purpose was to extend the use of ether anaesthesia beyond dentistry to major surgery, a project which was extremely bold at that time. Warren selected a patient who needed a tumour removed from his neck, and allowed Morton to anaesthetize the man with ether in an operating theatre where many eminent surgeons were gathered as spectators. The complete operation lasted about half an hour, and it was something of a lucky break for Morton that all went well, for his previous experience in dentistry had not involved very prolonged periods of anaesthesia. Apparently the patient was not wholly unconscious for this period, for although he reported feeling no pain, he said that he had experienced 'a sensation like that of scraping the part with a blunt instrument'. At the end of the operation, Warren pronounced the memorable words that are reported in so many medical histories: 'Gentlemen, this is no humbug!' thus distinguishing firmly between chemical anaesthesia and mesmerism, which the medical profession continued to regard as 'humbug'.

Morton's chief problem in seeking to patent and profit by the use of

ether for anaesthesia was that so common a substance was freely
available to anyone who cared to buy it. He therefore tried at first to
conceal the nature of his 'preparation' by masking its characteristic
smell by the addition of various aromatic essences. When Warren
planned to carry out further operations using Morton as an
anaesthetist, the medical fraternity objected that here was a technician
being employed who was using a *secret remedy*, a practice rightly
condemned by medical ethics. The Massachusetts Medical Society
ruled that drugs and other medical preparations should be freely
revealed to the world for the good of humanity. In order to compel
Morton to reveal the nature of his secret preparation, they forbade
Warren to perform any more operations with him until he abandoned
his secrecy.

There followed a dramatic incident in which a woman patient had
to wait outside the operating theatre at the Massachusetts General
Hospital, not knowing whether her leg was going to be amputated by
the usual method of strapping her down and ignoring her screams, or
of anaesthetizing her and performing the operation painlessly.
Elsewhere in the hospital the doctors were arguing with Morton and
offering him the alternatives of revealing the nature of the preparation
he proposed to use, or packing his bag and going. The extent to which
Morton's final decision was determined by the awful fate awaiting the
patient, or the sad fate awaiting his plans for becoming a medical
anaesthetist if he refused to divulge his secret, is a matter of differing
opinion among biographers. Morton did reveal his secret, admitting
that the scented, aromatic essences he had added to the ether were
quite redundant.

The details of this second and more serious operation performed
under ether are important in that they provide evidence regarding the
medical attitude to pain and anaesthesia which was to develop
throughout the civilized world. The operation of amputation was
entirely successful, and the patient afterwards testified that she felt no
pain; indeed, she awoke from the anaesthetic unaware that the
amputation had been accomplished. However, it is recorded that 'Just
as Warren was finishing Alice Mohan groaned, turning her head from
side to side.'[25] Thus, although all the observers accepted Alice
Mohan's subjective testimony that she felt no pain, they witnessed her
physical contortions and heard groans which are normally indicative
of pain. Furthermore, the doctors decided to accept that chemical
anaesthesia was 'genuine', whereas the majority of them stoutly
maintained that mesmeric anaesthesia was 'humbug'. Had they
witnessed a patient writhing and groaning under mesmeric anaesthesia
they would certainly have disbelieved her later testimony that she had
felt no pain.

The aura of mesmerism hangs over the early research into chemical anaesthesia. Morton and others noted that the attitudes and the personality of the patient were an important factor in determining how he would respond to ether; although they did not develop the idea, they recognized that pain is not a phenomenon that is wholly physiological in nature, but essentially a psychological experience. The basic personality of the patient is an important factor in determining how he will respond not only to mesmeric techniques but also to drugs. In these early days there was always the suspicion that the administration of gases was just a piece of flummery to impress the patient – just as Mesmer had used a *baquet*, a wand and soft music – and that in reality the anaesthetists were really mesmerizing their patients. Those conservative elements who dismissed mesmerism as 'humbug' were naturally prone to extend their scepticism to the anaesthesia induced by the administration of gases. Later in history, when the medical profession were converted to reliance on the pharmacological properties of the chemical anaesthetics, the anaesthetists were to condemn mesmeric and hypnotic techniques in surgery as quackery. It is only in very recent years that anaesthetists and other researchers into the problems of pain have begun coolly to consider the possibilities of hypnosis.

Because the practice of mesmerism was not allowed in most European and American hospitals, the medical mesmerists founded their own institutions. In the memorable year of 1846, when surgery was first performed under ether by Dr Warren, Elliotson took steps to found a mesmeric hospital in London; the London Mesmeric Infirmary was established at No. 9, Bedford Street in 1850. Later, mesmeric institutions were started in Bristol, Exeter and Dublin. So the coming of chemical anaesthesia did not supersede mesmeric anaesthesia entirely. At his Mesmeric Hospital in India, Esdaile is reported to have used a highly inefficient ether apparatus, but to have preferred the use of mesmerism.[26] At the Exeter Mesmeric Institute, J. B. Parker reported that he had 'performed upwards of two hundred surgical operations without the patients feeling pain, whilst under the influence of mesmerism, including twenty most painful operations on the eye'.[27]

It is interesting to speculate why the mesmeric doctors continued to rely on obtaining analgesia and anaesthesia by means of mesmerism when the chemical means of ether, and then chloroform, became readily available. As has been noted, whether a mesmeric trance can be induced depends very much on the personality of the patient, and even then it may take several hours of intensive work to induce a trance sufficiently deep to make an operation possible. Possibly the persistence of the mesmeric doctors can be attributed to the very human quality of cussedness: they were determined to demonstrate that they were not the charlatans their critics alleged them to be. Eventually, however, they lost heart and gave up, and with the collapse of the public faith in mesmerism, and acceptance of the reliability of chemical anaesthesia, mesmerism appeared to lose its power over patients, as Elliotson was later forced to admit.[28]

It is interesting to compare the rejection of the claim that mesmeric analgesia was genuine, with acceptance of the genuineness of the phenomenon when induced by pharmacological means, an acceptance which was accorded quite soon after Warren's historic operation in Boston in 1846. If one wished to argue the point, one could raise many of the objections put forward by such modern critics as T.X. Barber to acceptance of the reality of analgesia obtained by hypnotic suggestion, and contend that in most cases of chemical anaesthesia the patient only *pretends* not to feel pain.[29] Such a contention would appear quite absurd in the modern world, for we have grown up to believe in the reality of chemical anaesthesia; nevertheless, the matter is not quite as simple as it first appears, and it will be fruitful to discuss it further in later chapters.

The story of how Morton tried to get it accepted that he was the originator of anaesthesia by ether, and how Jackson claimed that the idea was his, Morton acting only under his instructions, is a long one. The United States Congress was prepared to make a grant of 100,000 dollars to the discoverer of so great a boon to humanity, and when the nature of this grant became generally known, a number of claimants came forward. Horace Wells was one, for although his efforts in dentistry had ended in partial failure, he had at least demonstrated the practicability of anaesthesia, using nitrous oxide, in 1844. Of the other claimants, some had indeed used ether successfully as an anaesthetic before Morton introduced it to Warren, but they had neither published their results nor systematically developed the practice. Among the contenders were Dr Crawford Long of Jefferson, Georgia, who had certainly used ether anaesthesia in 1842, and Dr E. E. Marcy of Hartford, who had operated with ether anaesthesia in 1845.

When it became plain that no one person could legitimately claim to be the originator of anaesthesia by gaseous inhalation, Congress decided that the prize could not be awarded. Morton and Jackson, at the height of their angry dispute, were jointly awarded a prize of 5,000 francs by the French *Académie des Sciences*.[30]

In 1846 and 1847 ether anaesthesia spread rapidly throughout the civilized world. Ether was not only used as an inhalant, but the Russian doctor N. I. Pigoroff demonstrated how ether vapour could successfully produce anaesthesia when injected into the rectum. Numerous gases were then tried to see if they were superior to ether; acetone, ethylene, benzene, chloroform, ACE (alcohol, chloroform and ether) and even coal gas had their advocates. Doctors everywhere knew all about gaseous anaesthesia in theory, but they were obviously waiting for somebody else to begin to apply it for fear of attracting opprobrium to themselves if things went wrong.

In 1849, Thomas Nunnely is reported to have examined thirty-seven compounds as possible anaesthetic agents.[31] The first alternative gas to ether which became popular was chloroform, and it was used extensively by the Scottish obstetrician James Young Simpson. He had initially tried ether, but found that many mothers objected to it on the grounds that it irritated the lungs.

Chloroform is actually a more dangerous and toxic gas than ether, but it has a pleasanter smell. Its anaesthetic properties had been known for some time, although in this era of medical conservatism and timidity, no one had dared to use it in clinical practice. Dr Simpson, having satisfied himself of its safety by inhaling it himself and testing it on a small group of colleagues, proceeded to use it in obstetric practice in 1847. This was a significant step forward in medicine, because although the battle for anaesthesia might be said to have been won when the conservative elements acquiesced in anaesthesia for the 'unnatural' pain of surgery, Simpson was using it for quite a different purpose, to combat the 'natural' pain of childbirth. This raised issues held to be crucial at the time.

Simpson's use of chloroform in childbirth was a landmark in the changing attitudes towards pain. Not only did many doctors oppose its use in such a field, but the Scottish clergy saw fit to make an issue of it. One clergyman pointed out that chloroform was simply another intoxicant like alcohol (which is perfectly true) and drew a picture of the lying-in room being turned into a scene of a drunken debauch every time a child was brought into the world! Another clergyman announced that 'Chloroform is a decoy of Satan, apparently offering itself to bless women; but in the end it will harden society and rob God of the deep, earnest cries which arise in time of trouble for help.'[32]

The comparison between chemical anaesthesia to avoid pain, and getting dead drunk on alcohol for precisely the same purpose, is a perfectly valid one. Society had long formulated moral views regarding the propriety or otherwise of drunkenness, and there is no special reason for discriminating between gin and chloroform as chemical agents, except that the latter is more efficient and controllable in its results. Even so, the medical profession have always been sensitive on the issue, and up to the 1930s the National Temperance Hospital in London would not allow alcohol in any form, even as a cleaning agent, to be used on its premises.

Simpson enjoyed controversy, and amused himself for some time at the expense of the clergy. His paper *Answers to the Religious Objection Against the Employment of Anaesthetic Agents in Midwifery and Surgery*[33] is a clever exercise in the use of biblical texts to refute the clerical objections. He also amused himself at the expense of a Dr Charles D. Meegs, a Philadelphia doctor who had originally criticized the Boston doctors for their introduction of ether anaesthesia. When Simpson addressed the clergy, he used dead-pan seriousness and scholarly erudition, but with Meegs he used barbed and outrageous ridicule.

The issue of pain in childbirth, which Simpson so insistently dragged into the arena of medical controversy, came to the forefront of public attention in 1853. In April of that year Queen Victoria elected to have chloroform for the birth of her seventh baby. This decision had a profound effect on the public acceptance of anaesthesia for childbirth.

In the controversy that followed, opponents of anaesthesia stressed the dangers of using chloroform, rather than its intoxicating effects. In fact, although chloroform, like other anaesthetic agents, is very occasionally fatal, the rate of maternal mortality was likely to be reduced rather than increased by sparing women some part of the pain of labour.

Queen Victoria's seventh accouchement took place under the direction of Sir James Clark, with Dr John Snow administering chloroform. A month later it was the subject of an editorial in *The Lancet*, which, astonishingly, denied that she had been anaesthetized. The statement began:

A very extraordinary report has obtained general circulation connected with the recent accouchment of her most gracious Majesty Queen Victoria. It was always been understood by the profession that the births of the Royal children in all instances have been unattended by any peculiar or untoward circumstances. Intense astonishment, therefore, has been excited throughout the profession by the rumour that her Majesty during her last labour was placed under the influence of chloroform, an agent which has unquestionably caused instantaneous death in a considerable number of cases. . . . On inquiry . . . we were not at all surprised to learn that in her late confinement the Queen was not rendered insensible by chloroform or by any other anaesthetic agent.[34]

This was a most disingenuous statement by the Editor. The last sentence reveals the policy that was adopted by the Palace in dealing with inquiries. It was reported that the Queen was *'not rendered insensible'*. Snow had no reluctance in admitting that he had administered chloroform to her, but it was maintained that she was never anaesthetized deeply enough to be called 'insensible'. This prevarication assisted the avoidance of the threat of scandal, but the public soon knew perfectly well that the Queen had demanded chloroform. Before the end of the year the term *anesthésie à la Reine* was in general use, and women were demanding chloroform for their confinements.[35] Dr Robert Lee, a violent opponent of analgesia for women in childbirth, attempted a counter-attack in a paper to the Royal Medical and Chirurgical Society in December of that year. He claimed to have accumulated records of seventeen cases in which chloroform had been used in labour with disastrous or fatal results, but the nearest he dared approach an attack on the Queen herself was to state that:

> Conceited or ignorant women of fashion made a passtime of this as of other quackeries, and the cause of science and humanity was placed in the hands of the most presumptuous and frivolous part of the community, while young and inexperienced mothers were decoyed to their destruction.[36]

Reformulation of Attitudes to Pain

The mid nineteenth century saw the creation of a new type of doctor, the anaesthetist, whose specialism it was to prevent pain. No such specialist had emerged before in the long history of medicine; the nearest had been the apothecary, who knew more about the prevention of pain than the physician or the surgeon. The first full-time anaesthetist in America was William Morton, a dentist, and because it was decided that the medical profession should pre-empt the craft of anaesthesia, they awarded Morton an honorary doctorate of medicine. In Britain, the first full-time anaesthetist was Dr John Snow, a London doctor who had gained his first anaesthetic experience not in surgery, but in administering ether to dental patients at St George's Hospital outpatients' clinic. With the coming of this new specialism in medicine, a new challenge was made to previous attitudes towards pain. The introduction of such chemical agents as local anaesthetics, analgesics, a huge variety of synthetic inhalants, and finally the psychotropic drugs, has been part of the vast growth of the pharmacological industry over the course of time.

The public grew to expect, to demand, that pain should be outlawed, and that it was up to their doctors to achieve this ambitious aim. Pressurized by patients on the one hand and by drug companies on the other, the medical profession developed a deep uneasiness on the issue of pain, by reason of the fact that the public demand was wholly Utopian. Doctors soon realized that the public must not be encouraged to think that they had a right to a pain-free existence. The barbarities of pain on the operating table could be abolished by anaesthesia, but it was dangerous to encourage the public to expect much more. This attitude was of course passed on to the new profession which developed under the medical aegis towards the end of the century, the nurses.

In the twentieth century, the problem of pain and its prevention has become the concern of a wide variety of specialists outside the medical profession. One of the most influential modern theories of pain which has had a widespread influence on clinical treatment, is the outcome of collaboration between a psychologist and a neurophysiologist, the gate control theory of Melzack and Wall.[37] The ironic paradox is that the great and progressive movement for the acceptance of chemical anaesthesia had to make its way in the mid nineteenth century by firmly repudiating those who knew most about the psychological aspects of pain, the mesmerists – with all their occult confusion and involvement with every sort of parapsychological nonsense. It was necessary firmly to insist on the *physiological* nature of pain and that its remedy lay entirely within the province of pharmacology, and later, surgery. In modern times the most forward-looking researchers are reconsidering the whole position and, as demonstrated at their symposia and conferences, somewhat regretting our comparative ignorance of mechanisms which the mesmerists were at least concerned with in their unscientific way. To quote a modern text by Merskey and Spear:

What repeatedly complicates the problem is a natural, but in our view mistaken, tendency for the word 'pain' to be used, particularly by doctors, to describe physical events. We are uncompromising in the view that this is not acceptable and that the word 'pain' is best used to refer to a psychological state. Of course we frequently imply, and readily agree, that there is much interesting and valuable information about some of the physical processes which are the counterpart of these events which we experience as pain; but we are insistent in our claim that physical changes which accompany or provoke such experiences are not, themselves, pain.[38]

REFERENCES

1 J. Priestley, *Experiments and Observations on Different Kinds of Air*, London: 1775.

2 H. Davy, *Researches, Chemical and Philosophical, Chiefly Concerning Nitrous Oxide* (1800), Facsimile Edition, London: Butterworths, 1972, pp. 465–556.

3 Ibid., pp. 538–9.

4 Ibid. S. T. Coleridge quoted, pp. 516–7.

5 B. McQuitty, *The Battle for Oblivion*, London: G. G. Harrap & Co., 1969, p. 36.

6 S. Wilks and G. T. Bettany, *A Biographical History of Guy's Hospital*, London: Ward, Lock, Bowden & Co., 1892, pp. 388–9.

7 See N. P. Rice, *Trials of a Public Benefactor as Illustrated in the Discovery of Etherization*, New York: Pudney & Russell, 1858, p. 82.

8 M. Faraday, 'Effects of inhaling the vapours of sulphuric ether', *Quarterly Journal of Science and the Arts*, 1818, 4, pp. 158–9.

9 'A forgotten pioneer of anaesthesia: Henry Hill Hickman, *British Medical Journal*, 13 April, 1912, p. 843.

10 For an account of the resuscitation of Anna Green after hanging, see E. S. Ellis, *Ancient Anodynes*, London: Heinemann, 1946, p. 11.

11 See *British Medical Journal*, 12 April, 1930, pp. 713–4.

12 T. E. Keys, *The History of Surgical Anaesthesia*, op. cit.

13 J. T. Gwathmey (ed.) *Anaesthesia*, op. cit.

14 F. H. Garrison, *An Introduction to the History of Medicine*, op. cit.

15 See N. E. Williams, 'The role of drug therapy', in S. Lipton (ed.), *Persistent Pain: Modern Methods of Treatment*, London: Academic Press, 1977.

16 E. S. Ellis, *Ancient Anodynes*, op. cit.

17 See G. C. Drew, W. P. Colquhoun and H. A. Long, 'Effect of small doses of alcohol on a skill resembling driving', *MRC Memorandum No. 38*, HMSO, 1959.

18 Burroughs, Wellcome & Co., *Anaesthetics Antient and Modern*, op. cit., p. 18.

19 See H. M. Lyman, *Artificial Anaesthesia and Anaesthetics*, New York: W. Wood & Co. 1881, p. 6.

20 Poster reproduced by B. McQuitty, *The Battle for Oblivion*, op. cit., Chap. IV.

21 See E. Andrews, 'The oxygen mixture; a new anaesthetic combination', *Chicago Medical Examiner*, 1868, 9, pp. 656–61.

22 T. E. Keys, *The History of Surgical Anaesthesia*, op. cit.

23 Cited by L. J. Ludovici, *Cone of Oblivion*, London: Max Parrish, 1961, p. 94.

24 E. W. Morton, 'The discovery of anaesthesia', *McClure's Magazine*, September 1896.

25 B. McQuitty, *The Battle for Oblivion*, op. cit., p. 92.

26 See *Report of the Mesmeric Hospital*, 'Record of the cases treated in the Mesmeric Hospital from June to December, 1847, with reports of the official visitors', Calcutta: W. Risdale, Military Orphan Press, 1848.

27 V. Robinson, *Victory Over Pain*, op. cit., p. 76.

28 See G. Rosen, 'From mesmerism to hypnotism', *Ciba Symposium*, 1948, 9, pp. 838–44.

29 See T. X. Barber, *LSD, Marihuana, Yoga and Hypnosis*, Chicago: Aldine Publishing Co., 1970, Chap. 5.

30 Académie des Sciences, *Compte Rendu*, 1847, p. 24.

31 See A. B. Luckhardt, 'Ethylene anaesthesia', in J. T. Gwathmey (ed.), *Anaesthesia*, op. cit.

32 Cited by H. W. Haggard, *Devils, Drugs and Doctors*, op. cit., p. 108.

33 Cited by W. O. Priestley and H. R. Storer (eds), *The Obstetric Memoirs and Contributions of James Y. Simpson*, Philadelphia: J. B. Lippincott & Co., 1856.

34 Editorial, *The Lancet*, 14 May, 1853, p. 453.

35 See Herbert Thoms, '"Anesthésie à la Reine", a chapter in the history of anaesthesia', *American Journal of Obstetrics and Gynecology*, 1940, 40, pp. 340–6.

36 R. Lee, 'An account of 17 cases of parturition in which chloroform was inhaled with pernicious effects', *American Journal of Obstetrics and Gynecology*, 17 December, 1853, pp. 608–11.

37 R. Melzack and P. D. Wall, 'Pain mechanisms: A new theory', *Science*, 1965, 150, pp. 971–9.

38 H. Merskey and F. G. Spear, *Pain: Psychological and Psychiatric Aspects*, op. cit., pp. vii–viii.

3

THE NATURE OF PAIN

Neuroanatomy and Physiology

Before we proceed to discuss theories of the nature of pain, it is necessary to outline the elements of the anatomy and function of the nervous system. Although, as already stated, this book presents a psychological rather than a neurophysiological approach to the problem of pain, a basic knowledge of the human nervous system is essential to the understanding of some of the theories discussed. The scientifically sophisticated reader will, of course, have no need to read this preamble which, for the sake of brevity, presents a picture which is over-simplified.

Nerves serve two purposes, and are accordingly specialized. *Motor* nerves carry messages down from the brain to stimulate the muscles; *sensory* nerves carry messages inwards from the periphery (skin, sense organs, viscera, etc.) to inform the brain of what is going on in all parts of the body. Outgoing neural impulses are referred to as 'efferent', and incoming impulses as 'afferent'; these terms are often applied to the nerves themselves. Where nerve trunks occur in the body they are rather like telephone cables containing a bundle of wires; the nerve trunks contain fibres of both motor and sensory nerves running alongside one another in the same conduit. Most of the nerves in the body are not connected directly with the brain; instead, they go to the nearest segment of the spinal cord which is contained in the bony tube of the backbone. There are some exceptions to this; for instance, the nerves of the head (cranial nerves) go directly into openings in the skull.

Although both motor and sensory nerves often lie alongside one another in the same nerve trunk, close to the spine they are divided, the motor nerves to the front (ventral root) and the sensory nerves to the back (dorsal root), before they join the neural cord within. The basic difference between the functions of the two types of nerves, motor and sensory, was discovered by a Scottish physiologist and surgeon, Charles Bell, in the early part of the nineteenth century. Thus, if the motor root of a nerve trunk is severed where it emerges from the spine, the patient will lose control of his muscles in the relevant part of his body; but if the sensory root is cut, he will lose most of the sensation from that part.

Nerve fibres are made up of greatly elongated cells. At one end there is the cell body containing the cell nucleus, from one side of which there projects a branch known as the *axon*, which may be anything up to three feet in length in the human. Also projecting from the cell body are a large number of short fibres, the *dendrites*. The whole assemblage of cell body, axon and dendrites is known as a *neuron*.

Although the axons which make up the nerve fibres may be very long, the neurons which make up most of the brain tissue may be only a few thousandths of an inch long. Typically, neurons communicate with one another by sending impulses from the cell body along the axon to make contact with the dendrites of other cells, such contact being known as a *synapse*. Thus information about a touch on the hand is not conveyed to the upper part of the brain along one continuous nerve, but through a series of synapses, the first synaptic junction occurring where the sensory nerve joins the spinal cord. The system may be thought of by analogy with a series of electrical relays in a circuit, but too much must not be made of this electrical analogy. Neural impulses travel very much more slowly than an electric current, and the rate of travel of impulses varies greatly with the thickness of the axon; in thin axons the rate of travel may be only about a yard a second, whereas in thick axons the rate may be a hundred times faster.

When one neuron communicates with another the effect may be excitatory or inhibitory: that is, the axon of neuron A may excite the dendrites of neuron B so that the cell body of the latter 'fires'; alternatively the stimulation may be of such a nature that B is rendered strongly resistant to firing even though it receives some positive excitation from elsewhere. The different rates of conductance in different types of nerve fibres, combined with the fact that some impulses have a positive, excitatory function, and others an inhibitory function, have important implications for the complexity of the total impression of the nature of events which are happening to our bodies conveyed to our consciousness by the sensory nervous system.

The simple picture so far conveyed is that sensory nerves arise as minute branches in the skin and other sentient tissues, and travel to the spinal cord (except in the case of the cranial nerves) in nerve trunks, entering the cord by the dorsal root. Within the cord, by a process of repeated synapses, neural impulses are conveyed up to various parts of the brain, which is a great mass of tissue largely composed of neural networks specialized for various functions.

The impulses which are conveyed to the muscles travel in the opposite direction. Arising within the brain, they travel by a series of synapses down the spinal cord, out at the ventral root and along the motor nerves to the muscles. Since impulses may have an excitatory or an inhibitory function, the efferent impulses may cause muscles either to contract or to relax. The brain is not always involved in the actions of the body; some of the simple muscular mechanisms are co-ordinated at a spinal level. This is demonstrated by the fact that a decapitated chicken may be able to run about for a few moments.

The brain of all higher animals has evolved on the same basic pattern, but according to the habits of the animal species the anatomy is different. Thus the dogfish, which is dependent on hunting by smell, has large olfactory lobes in the brain. Birds which have complex flight patterns have a specially well-developed *cerebellum*, the part of the brain concerned with balance and integration of muscular movement. The human species, with its greater intellectual powers, has a greatly enlarged *cerebral cortex*. Basically, however, the brain of all higher animals consists of three parts, the primitive *central core*, the 'old brain' (*limbic system*) and the 'new brain' (*cerebral cortex*); the names of the latter two sections refer to oldness and newness in evolutionary development.

Where the spinal cord enters the skull it enlarges to form the brain stem and central core. The upper part of this core is known as the *thalamus*, which may be compared to an elaborate telephone switchboard. Afferent impulses which come up the spinal cord are relayed there to various other parts of the brain, and efferent impulses from various sites of the brain are relayed elsewhere, some of them passing down the cord. The 'old brain' is concerned with many automatic functions, such as control of digestion and circulation, and is therefore sometimes known as the *visceral brain*. The 'new brain' is the part which processes what we regard as 'thinking', and is the seat of conscious control and experience. To some extent there is localization of function in the 'new brain'; thus there are definite areas which appear to be related to feeling in different parts of the body, and again, definite areas associated with control of specific muscle groups. These areas have been mapped with considerable precision by surgeons operating on the brains of conscious patients (using a local anaesthetic for the sentient tissue) and stimulating different points of the cortex electrically.[1] This establishment of topographical structure does not mean that relevant sensations from, and control of, particular parts of the body are *wholly* vested in special cortical areas; on the contrary, a simple stimulus has representations in various parts of the brain, and a simple action likewise involves the co-ordination of afferent impulses from various sites.

For the purpose of studying pain, particular attention must be paid to a structure within the brain known as the *reticular formation*. This is a mesh of neurons, about the size of one's little finger, which lies within the central core of the brain. It sends relay fibres to the various parts of the brain above it, and other fibres down the spinal cord. The function of the reticular formation is that of an arousal system, and the general action of sleep and of anaesthetic drugs is to dampen it down. Thus in the sleeping or anaesthetized person stimuli still arrive at the cerebral cortex, but no reaction is produced because of the quiescence of the reticular formation.

Melzack makes the point that our actual knowledge of what goes on in the brain is rather limited, and a matter of inference rather than proven fact. Writing of the arrival of afferent stimuli, associated with the experience of pain, at the thalamus and reticular formation, he says:

> Factual information about the afferent processes related to pain really ends at this point. We know that nerve impulses are projected to the cortex but, because large cortical lesions rarely diminish or abolish pain, it is assumed that the cortical projections represent only one of several pathways involved in pain. Other pathways project to the limbic system that forms an extensive and important part of the brain. Moreover, there is evidence that the cortex is not a final destination (or 'pain centre') but that it processes the information it receives and transmits it to deeper portions of the brain. In short, the afferent process from skin to cortex marks only the beginning of prolonged, interacting activities.[2]

The reader is warned that the brief account given in this chapter is a very oversimplified picture of the nervous system; nevertheless, it contains enough of the basic principles of neuroanatomy and physiology to make what follows more comprehensible to the layman who has no knowledge of these matters. This account has omitted all mention of a separately organized nervous system which controls many functions of the animal body, the *autonomic system*. This lies entirely outside the brain and spinal cord (together known as the *central nervous system* – CNS). Autonomic nerves synapse with the spinal roots of the other nervous system, and thus the whole body mechanism is harmonized. The autonomic system is concerned with self-regulatory activities of the body such as sweating, digestion and control of the pupil size in the eye, which are not under our voluntary control. Beyond mentioning its existence, and the fact that it has two divisions, sympathetic and parasympathetic, which are concerned with promoting contrasting body changes (changes related to violent activity versus passive, relaxing activity) the nature of the autonomic nervous system need not be discussed further at this point.

A final point regarding the ability of the nervous system to perceive pain concerns the chemical substances secreted by the body which are known as *endorphins* and *enkephalins*. Study of these substances is so recent that mention of them does not occur in books and articles prior to 1975, and acknowledgement of their existence has radically advanced our understanding of the mechanisms of pain. The pace of discovery of facts about these chemical substances is so rapid that anything now published about them will be a little outmoded in a few years' time.

For some time it had been known that the brain contains special *receptor sites* which are sensitive to the action of opioid drugs like morphine which kill pain. A consideration of this fact gave the strange impression that the Almighty, when he was designing Adam on the drawing-board, planned certain structures in the neural tissue whose sole function it was to respond to the products of the opium poppy when the descendants of Adam had got round to manufacturing them and eating them. A less fanciful supposition was that in certain circumstances the body itself produces chemicals that are chemically similar to the opium products and whose function it is to damp down pain. The principle of dual control of behaviour and experience by nervous and chemical means is typical of many body systems.

The 'keyholes' in the neural tissue in the form of receptor sites having been found, it remained to discover the natural chemical 'keys' to fit them. Obviously such 'keys' had to be somewhat similar to the opioid drugs chemically, as the latter seem to fit the 'keyholes'. It is not proposed in this account to discuss the chemical nature of the substances discovered, but merely to note their existence. Various laboratories in the early 1970s were trying to identify the relevant substances among the many glandular secretions found in the brain, and in 1974 Hughes and Kosterlitz[3] at the University of Aberdeen isolated from animal brain tissue chemical substances known as *enkephalins*, which were similar in action and chemical structure to morphine. Research workers in other laboratories also advanced this new and important study, and Eric Simon of New York University coined the generic name *endorphins*, from end(ogenous) (m)orphines, to cover a range of naturally occurring secretions which have a morphine-like action.

An interesting aspect of this work is the discovery of morphine antagonists, such as *naloxone*, which counteract the effect of morphine, and of the naturally occurring endorphins and enkephalins. (If someone is suffering from an overdose of morphine he may be resuscitated by the injection of naloxone.) Naloxone functions by competing successfully for the receptor sites within the neural tissue, 'binding' with them and rendering them unresponsive to morphine and to the body's own opioids. This has an important use in research, for in an animal laboratory if it is supposed that a procedure renders animals analgesic by virtue of their internal secretion of endorphins and enkephalins, injection of naloxone will prove a crucial test because of its power to cancel the opioid action. As described in a later chapter, this naloxone test was used with human subjects to investigate whether the analgesia induced by suggestion under hypnosis was due to the secretion of endorphins and enkephalins.

Pain and Pleasure

It is natural to suppose that every living creature has mechanisms which, when activated, will inform it of harmful events in the environment. Or, to put it another way, that when an animal is jabbed or otherwise damaged, the jab will send a 'message of pain' to the brain. This assumption is rather too simple; the survival and general efficiency of even quite lowly creatures could not be maintained by such an arrangement. It is more realistic to think of the animal simultaneously maintaining its defences and maximizing its over-all well-being by a rather more sophisticated arrangement. On the one hand it is constantly and actively *looking out for trouble*; on the other hand it is actively scanning the environment, looking for *sources of pleasure and profit*. Whether a jab is perceived as pain, or pleasure, or not perceived at all, depends on past experience, present anticipation, current emotional state and understanding of the total present situation.

In some circumstances it may be of advantage for an animal to be aggressive and press home an attack, utterly undeterred by such wounds as it incurs in the process. Even the mild rabbit needs to fight with tooth and claw when protecting its young or competing for a mate. In an emergency it would be disadvantageous to be inhibited by the experience of pain. Some humans confess to sometimes enjoying a 'punch-up'; the giving and receiving of blows is then a positive pleasure. In other circumstances, when flight is the best policy, the experience of acute pain attendant on receiving even a scratch, will strongly motivate the fleeing animal.

It used to be thought (and indeed is still taught by some old-fashioned textbooks) that the skin and other organs contain 'pain receptors', that is, specialized ends of nerves which when stimulated would send messages of pure pain to the brain. This conclusion was drawn, understandably, when very high-powered microscopes came into use in the nineteenth century, and the minute structure of the skin could be examined. There is a great variety of end organs to be seen in the skin, from which the fibres of sensory nerves originate. It was natural to assume that some of these were specialized to detect pressure, heat, cold or pain. The older textbooks of physiology give elaborate details of the functions of the specialized receptors, with considerable confidence. This concept, known as 'specificity theory', was based on the physiological work of Charles Bell and the later work of Magendie. It was elaborated towards the end of the nineteenth century by such writers as Weber, Von Frey and Schiff,[4] and replaced the older assumption that pain was merely a greatly *intensified* stimulus of touch, heat or cold.

A question which is never answered in the old textbooks is the following: If there are fibres conveying 'impulses of pain', where are the fibres conveying 'impulses of pleasure'? Some people may find such a question disturbing, and try to deflect it by maintaining that not only are pain and pleasure unalike in quality, but unalike in nature. As some readers may feel that they are being side-tracked from a very important question, it is necessary to discuss the philosophical background of this question.

St Thomas Aquinas distinguished between carnal pleasures, which came from the senses, and the pleasures of the mind. He wrote:

> There are two phases in pleasure: the perception of what is congenial, which belongs to cognition, and the satisfaction in what is offered, which belongs to the appetite, where desire culminates.[5]

Aquinas believed that both pain and pleasure depended upon the senses, but that the 'operation' of the mind was necessary for their creation. He wrote in the tradition of Aristotle, as did Descartes, who in his *Traité de les Passions de l'Âme* regarded both pain and pleasure as indefinable epiphenomena of the bodily events which the mind perceives. Spinoza followed Descartes to the extent that he continued to treat pain not as a sense like touch or vision, but as an emotion like melancholy and dolor. Although Descartes agreed with Aristotle that pain was 'a passion of the soul', he nevertheless proposed a rather simple model of how the mind was appraised of physical events which led to this passion being generated. In his *L'Homme*[7] he gives a diagram of a human figure whose foot is being burnt by a spark from a fire; it shows the neural pathway by which awareness of the event is conveyed to the brain, to the pineal gland and thence to the incorporeal soul.

The mechanistic part of Descartes' theory was to be very influential in the succeeding centuries, and when nineteenth-century scientists left the incorporeal soul out of their considerations, the epiphenomenal nature of Descartes' and Spinoza's concept of pain was also rejected.

Pain came to be identified with the neural impulse itself.

The common view is, therefore, that whereas pain is an unpleasant
physical sensation, pleasure consists of a combination of a number of
sensations and an appreciation of the general circumstances. A fine
morning, a beautiful view, a refreshing swim and a carefree mind, all
these would contribute to a feeling of pleasure. In the common view,
we would not expect to find nerve fibres specifically concerned with
conveying sensations of pleasure. A girl may agree that the sensory
nerves with which her lips are so plentifully endowed convey the
pleasure of a kiss; yet although the physical stimulation is the same, the
kiss is pleasurable when given by an attractive man, but not when
given by an ugly old lecher. Pleasure is presumed to result from what
we do with the totality of our sensory experience. However, as we shall
see, the essential nature of pleasure and pain are more alike than is
generally supposed. The idea that pain is simply a sensation cannot
really be maintained in the face of all the evidence that will be
presented. This may be said notwithstanding the fact that many
textbooks of surgery, medicine and physiology still used by doctors,
dentists and students, bear chapters entitled 'Pain Sensation'.

The reality is that just as there are no specific nerves of pleasure, so
there are no specific nerves of pain. The same neural pathways can
give us an experience of pleasure or of pain depending on a host of
complex factors, including the rate and intensity of neural firing, the
relative degree of stimulation in parallel neural pathways, our past
experience and our interpretation of the whole circumstances of our
receiving the stimuli. Pleasure and pain are both *psychological*
experiences.

It is often difficult to convince the average person of the essentially
psychological nature of pain. Jab him with a pin and he is likely to say,
'Damn my psyche – that was entirely a matter of my soma!' He may
agree that some pains – the pain of bereavement, the agony of despair
and depression – are psychological, but, he maintains, although it is
not easy precisely to define how they differ from crude physical pain,
they are somehow 'pains' of a different sort. He may stoutly declare
that the result of physical damage is not primarily a psychological
experience, but an entirely physical sensation. Indeed, the average
medical practitioner, reared in the traditions of twentieth-century
medicine, will thoroughly agree with this layman's commonsense view
of pain. It is only when he encounters patients who appear to have
nothing wrong with them organically, yet are in constant pain, that he
will have cause to wonder. Either he will admit that the conventional
medical view of pain needs considerable up-dating, or he will take
refuge in the view that his patients who appear to be physically sound,
although complaining bitterly of pain, have that variety of pain most

conveniently dismissed as 'hysterical'. This latter view is powerfully supported by the mythology which the Freudians have helped to foster, which maintains that some patients suffer because they 'want' or 'need' to suffer, and that the nature of a pain that the patient 'chooses' to have is symbolic of his predicament. Thus in the case of a patient, Frau Cäcilie M., Freud interpreted a facial neuralgia in terms of the lady having endured a humiliating scene which was 'a slap in the face' for her.[8] This way of reasoning provides the perfect let-out for the physician who is unable either to diagnose any cause of pain or to provide any effective treatment. The Freudian let-out absolves the doctor from the charge of personal incompetence, or from admitting that what he regards as medical science is inadequate in both theory and method.

It should be remarked in passing that the Freudian point of view, which stresses the motivational aspects of pain, will not be disregarded in this book. In particular, the views of one unorthodox Freudian writer, Thomas Szasz, as set out in his essay on *L'Homme Douloureux*,[9] will be considered.

The Semantic Trap

Although at the level of intellectual argument the reader may be prepared to grant that pain can more usefully be considered as a psychological experience than as a physical sensation, it is more likely that this basic point will meet with considerable reservation. The whole of our language, and hence our way of thinking, treats pain as if it were a sensation; semantics endorses a dualistic approach which insists that there is a fundamental difference between 'mind' and 'body'.

The fact that language has crystallized certain modes of thinking, has forced some of the foremost critics of the idea that pain is a sensation into a semantic trap. Thus in the course of a lecture, Barry Wyke said:

> Pain is not a sensory experience like vision, touch or kinaesthesia, it is an abnormal emotional state; and when a patient consults a clinician, it is relief from that disordered emotional state that the patient is seeking, and nothing else. . . . The perceptual experiences which accompany this disordered state are not the pain; what the patient tells you about in your consulting room is his emotional status. And this is why parametric measurement of reflex effects of EEG cannot tell you anything about the nature of this disordered emotional state. They are epiphenomena.[10]

This makes Wyke's own view clear enough (a point of view which is not entirely shared by the present author), yet later in the same lecture he was forced to fall back on the old terminology. In trying to describe the neurophysiological mechanisms which accompany normal function where there is slight but non-painful damage to tissues, he resorted to such expressions as 'the painful stimulus' as a shorthand for 'the-stimulus-which-would-be-painful-were-it-not-for-the-blocking-mechanism'. Indeed the term 'pain receptor', which owes its ancestry to the specificity theory of pain, was used by Wyke in arguing *against* this theory. The term 'pain receptor' implies that pain is something out there in the environment, like light and sound, which is reacted to at the periphery and sent in to some pain-registering centre in the brain. What can we do with terms like these that imply a whole body of outmoded theory? It seems best, before we pursue the argument further and consider the rival theories of pain in some detail, to look at certain puzzles and paradoxes in the study of pain, for they force us carefully to consider the adequacy of the views about pain with which we have grown up.

The Paradoxes of Pain

The paradoxes associated with pain are perfectly familiar to the average doctor and to many laymen; they provide convenient touchstones for assessing the validity of various alternative theories of pain. The first and perhaps best-known paradoxical condition is that of phantom pain. When patients have had a limb amputated their initial feeling is that the limb is still there because they continue to receive sensations which appear to come from out in space where the limb used to be. At first, the phantom limb seems to resemble a real one in both shape and size, and the patient may be haunted by the recurring impression that he can use it for its proper purpose. However, after a while this impression fades, and although the patient still has strange sensations, the phantom limb typically seems to telescope and to retreat into the stump.[11]

Pain in the phantom limb is reported by about 35 per cent of amputees,[12] but it fades and disappears in all but a small minority of patients, who are doomed to suffer some degree of chronic pain. The size of this minority (about 2 to 13 per cent in the various studies) depends upon the type of the patient population. The pain may have the horribly realistic feature of appearing to relate to the structure of a missing part, as when the fingers of a phantom hand appear to be cramping into a clenched fist.

Trouble with phantom limb pain may persist intermittently for years, despite the fact that the stump has healed perfectly.[13] Even when the pain in the phantom limb dies down, it can be reactivated by stimulation of 'trigger zones', areas of the body distant from the stump which somehow revive the aching. The phantom limb may become a veritable Achilles heel to the amputee, and years later any serious pain or psychological stress may revive his suffering. Cohen has described the onset of phantom limb pain in a patient who developed anginal pain twenty-five years after an amputation.[14]

It is difficult to account for this curious condition of pain. It is rarely associated with any abnormality in the healed stump, and attempts to stop it by dissecting out the outgrowths from the severed nerves (neuromas) in the stump are not very successful. Furthermore, there is the unsolved mystery of why some amputees suffer from this condition but most do not. Kolb[15] has suggested that those amputees who continue to suffer from painful phantoms are people who stubbornly cling to a body-image which they are reluctant to relinquish. Similarly, Szasz[16] maintains that the painful phantom is the result of the patient neurotically trying to deny to himself the loss of the limb. These typically Freudian speculations have been challenged by others such as Simmel,[17] who reports that in her considerable experience of this condition, the patients show full awareness of the unpleasant loss and its consequences. It is only when the phantom is in existence, but not painful, that patients may tend to deny its existence, for as Kolb points out, they may fear to be regarded as deranged for insisting on feeling something which is so obviously missing. There is some evidence that amputees who have phantom limb pain are no more neurotic by disposition than those who do not suffer from the syndrome, as shown by Ewalt et al. who studied 404 amputees, of whom only eight complained of phantom limb pain.[18]

Research has shown that the condition is less likely to occur where the severance of the limb has been sudden and accidental, for example with soldiers in battle. By contrast, where the amputation has taken place following a pathological and painful condition in some part of the limb which was endured for an appreciable time before amputation, the pain is likely to be perpetuated in the phantom. Thus a patient who had suffered badly from a splinter of wood beneath a finger-nail, and then lost his hand in an accident, experienced a phantom hand with a painful finger.[19] It seems, therefore, that a pre-amputation pain is somehow perpetuated as an on-going experience in the memory, and is referred to the phantom. This is all the more strange in view of the fact that we do not normally remember pain: we can certainly remember having had a painful experience, but the actual quality of the pain cannot be recalled. In the case of the person with the injured finger, if it had been allowed to heal normally the pain would have disappeared and been forgotten. It was only because the hand had been lost while the finger still hurt that the pain was somehow perpetuated 'in the mind'. When we say that the pain is 'in the mind', it is not suggested that an incorporeal ghost inhabits the physical organism. The limb is referred to as a phantom because there is no limb there to suffer, but the pain is best conceived as a percept arising from on-going activity in neural structures in the central nervous system, which was once initiated by the injury and is afterwards perpetuated in a manner which we frankly do not understand.

Another paradoxical pain condition is that of causalgia, which literally means 'burning pain'. This variety of pathological pain, which is experienced as scalding or scorching over an area of the skin, is typically the aftermath of the partial severance of a nerve trunk in some peripheral part of the body. The strange thing about the condition is that it begins some time after the injury has begun to heal. The burning pain is not continuous but may be triggered off by gentle stimulation, such as the skin being stroked, or by sudden noises, vibration or emotional upsets. Weir Mitchell, who, after treating wounds in the American Civil War, was one of the first adequately to document the condition, described causalgia as one of the most terrible pains that could be inflicted by a nerve wound.[20]

The study of causalgia reveals a most interesting fact about pain: that not only can it result from massive sensory input, as when a part is cut or crushed, but also from an *absence* of input. For what is lacking as a consequence of the type of injury producing causalgia is the normal sensory input from that part of the limb *beyond* (distal to) the site of the injury to the sensory nerve. In the brief discussion of neuroanatomy at the beginning of this chapter it was made clear that an injury to a sensory nerve trunk in, say, the upper arm may cut off parts of the forearm and hand from sending their normal messages to the brain. Gentle stroking of the skin will send sensory messages through other uninjured pathways, and it is because the total pattern of sensory input is *unbalanced* that the sense data which are received are processed in an abnormal manner and experienced as a terrible burning pain.

If we rap our thumb gently we experience a slight smart, but if we hit it hard we experience a strong pain. The idea therefore grew up that pain was merely a sensation of touch (or some other modality) of an extremely intense nature, and such simple-minded reasoning seems superficially plausible. However, the facts about phantom limb pain and causalgia plainly do not fit in with this concept.

Another condition, somewhat similar to causalgia, is post-herpetic neuralgia. Here there has been an attack on the nerve fibres in the skin by the virus *herpes zoster*, a virus similar to that which causes chickenpox. The viral attack (commonly known as 'shingles') causes some damage to the network of sensory nerves, and it is during the healing process that, in a minority of cases, the patient is subject to attacks of pain.

The 'shingles' are eruptions that plainly mark out an area of skin which has been attacked. The post-herpetic pain is not confined to these areas, and gentle stimulation, such as the friction of clothes, can bring on attacks of neuralgic pain which may last intermittently for many months or years. Here we have the same paradox as with causalgia; gentle stimulation produces massive pain, and it seems that the cause is probably similar.

This neuralgic condition also shows the phenomenon of *summation* in response to stimuli within the affected area. As Noordenbos[21] has demonstrated, the reaction to tactile or thermal stimulation may not be immediate. The application of repeated gentle pin-pricks, or of a test-tube full of hot water, does not immediately feel unpleasant to the patient; then, after a delay of as long as a minute, there is a sudden burst of pain. It is as though somewhere in the nervous system there is a build-up of energy as, by analogy, an electrical condenser accumulates a charge and then suddenly discharges. A further characteristic of the phenomenon of summation is that the time required for the pain reaction to occur is shorter in proportion to the size of the area of skin which is stimulated.

It has been suggested that in this condition the network of sensory nerves has been unevenly attacked, and that some fibres regenerate before others, so that the normal pattern of balanced sensory input is interfered with, and an astonishing degree of pain can be experienced from very mild stimuli. In a later study, Noordenbos[22] reported that the virus *herpes zoster* selectively attacks the different types of nerve fibres, with more of the large-diameter fibres being destroyed. The significance of this sort of imbalance in the generation of pain will be discussed later.

Another condition in which there may be selective loss of the larger nerve fibres is the *tic douloureux*, or trigeminal neuralgia. In this condition the alteration in the network of sensory nerves is presumed to be the result of an abnormal process of ageing rather than of viral attack.[23] This is a very distressing condition in which one side of the face is subject to paroxysms of severe pain. As with post-herpetic neuralgia, there is the same phenomenon of summation; repeated gentle touches at one trigger spot will set off a burst of pain after some delay, but more vigorous contact with the face may produce no result. The severe pain lasts for a short while and is then followed by a dull ache; there may then be no more pain for several minutes or hours.

A curious feature of the *tic douloureux* is that it may mysteriously remit for a matter of weeks or months, and then return for no apparent reason. In the past, patients with this condition were often suspected of malingering; doctors believed that the disorder was really hysterical, the condition being revived from time to time to suit the patient's convenience. The condition does not respond well to analgesic drugs by mouth, or to the injection of a local anaesthetic, so neurosurgery was sometimes resorted to. But even when nerves fibres carrying sensation from the face to the brain are severed, the *tic douloureux* can still continue. Strangely, the drug which was found to relieve it was one used in the treatment of epilepsy, Tegretol (carbamazipine). This drug acts directly on the brain, and its role in relieving this neuralgic condition suggests that once the disorder is established, the trouble is continued within the brain itself by a mechanism perhaps similar to that which is operative in phantom limb pain.

These examples of paradoxical pain have been cited at some length to make clear that the early concept of pain being no more than a sensation generated by damage to a receptor organ and carried to the brain along a 'pain fibre' is simply inadequate to account for the observable facts.

Theories of Pain

Specificity theory, which has been briefly outlined, provided the simple rationale for surgeons to attempt to terminate chronic pain by cutting through the nerve which was allegedly carrying the unwanted pain impulse, much as one might snip through a telephone wire to interrupt an unwanted message. As early as 1906 Sherrington[24] doubted the specificity of any pain receptor, and indeed many surgical procedures designed to interrupt the supposed pathways of the pain impulses have not been very successful.

Here we must make a distinction between *specialization of function* and *specificity*. Specialization in this context means that a neural structure is specialized so that it reacts only to a particular type of stimulus, but the neural impulses it engenders and sends up to the brain can be modulated by the information-processing system to produce a variety of experience (e.g. pain or pleasure). Specificity implies that a neural structure subserves only one type of experience, e.g. the optic nerve gives us the experience of vision, and vision only. Specificity theory assumed that pain was a discrete modality, comparable to vision, hearing, smell, etc.

In the 1890s, theories based on pattern recognition and central summation of neural impulses began to be developed by theorists such as Goldscheider.[25] Theories of pattern recognition obviated the necessity for postulating specific pain receptors, and suggested instead that pain resulted from the stimulation of multiple receptors. Such theories have found support in more modern times from neurophysiologists such as Weddell[26] and Livingston.[27] The latter has suggested that noxious stimuli activate structures within the spinal cord which send messages to the brain where they are interpreted in terms of temporal and spatial relationships, and thus build up into an experience of pain. Bishop[28] has suggested that the input to the structures within the spinal cord is modified by a mechanism under efferent control which may prevent summation from occurring. This introduces the important concept of relative degrees of readiness to perceive pain being controlled by higher centres of the brain. This general view was also proposed by Noordenbos[29] in the same year.

The various conditions of paradoxical pain which have been described above fit more readily into the more complex theory which recognizes the role of the brain in summating and processing the stimuli it receives before they are perceived as painful or not. When the modulating system becomes ineffective for various psychological reasons, then pain may be the end product of incoming stimuli which would normally be perceived as innocuous.

The most recent theory of the nature of pain is the gate control theory proposed by Melzack and Wall in 1965.[30] This further elaborates the theories of pattern recognition and central summation, and, in particular, proposes that there is a controlling 'gate mechanism' within the spinal cord, which is opened and closed to permit a greater or lesser volume of neural stimulation associated with pain to flow through it. This theory has been very influential in all subsequent research into pain mechanisms; although criticized on various technical points over the past seventeen years, it is still very robust, and has not been replaced by any rival theory. In 1976 Wall[31] updated it in a number of minor ways and answered critics.

Gate control theory originated in the collaboration between a psychologist (Melzack) and a neurophysiologist (Wall). The elements of the theory may be understood with reference to the diagram below. It is proposed that afferent neural impulses travel in from the periphery (skin, muscles, viscera, etc.) to the *transmission cells* (T cells) in the spinal cord, via that region of the cord known as the *substantia gelatinosa* (SG), where there is a modulating mechanism, or 'gate', which controls the volume of flow. The function of the T cells is to stimulate the action system.

It will be seen in the diagram that the input of neural impulses travels along two types of nerve fibres, having large and small diameters respectively. Both types stimulate the T cells to initiate action, but such action is inhibited to a greater or lesser degree by the

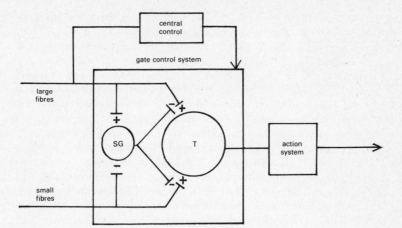

After R. Melzack and P. D. Wall (1965)[32]

activity of the SG. However, the effect of large and small fibres on the SG is contrary; the large fibres promote its inhibitory action (and hence close the 'gate'), whereas the small fibres decrease its inhibitory action, so that the 'gate' swings wide open.

A further mechanism is shown in the diagram; the large diameter fibres project up to the *central control* (i.e. the brain) which sends down feedback messages to the gate control system. Thus, not only is the state of the gate influenced by the stimuli arriving along sensory fibres of large and small diameter, but the state of affairs in the brain is exerting a control. Thus in a condition of anxiety when the animal is on the look-out for possible hurt, the brain causes the gate to open wide.

It is suggested that the nervous system is not inert until something jolts it, but that all the time there are naturally-occurring incoming stimuli, and that the small diameter fibres are constantly bombarding the spinal cord with relatively small impulses which serve to hold the gate open. This activity is balanced by stimuli coming in via the large diameter fibres which have a contrary influence. The reader can easily test this hypothesis by very gently giving the surface of his skin repeated pricks with a needle to stimulate the smallest nerve fibres; a tiny, sharp pain will arise; if he then rubs the area roughly to stimulate the large fibres, the pain will immediately disappear.

This, in brief, is a very simplified account of the mechanism which gate control theory postulates at the level of the spinal cord where sensory stimuli are received before being relayed up to the brain. This theory also states that stimuli arriving at the brain are conveyed to its various parts in a highly complex manner, the reticular system playing a key role both in arousing the higher centres and in sending down efferent stimuli which affect the control of the postulated gate mechanism.

It must not be thought that gate control theory has received universal acceptance. Many eminent authorities working in the clinical field and in experimental pain research were antagonistic towards the new theory. Thus in 1972 Schmidt[33] expressed his scepticism of its usefulness and referred to it as an 'unlikely hypothesis'; his opposition was supported, in the same collection of papers, by Iggo. According to Wall, 'A welcome 19th century virulence appeared in the literature'[34]; he has also referred to the spirited defences of the 'Old Believers', indicating the Thirteenth Edition of Mountcastle's *Medical Physiology* (1974),[35] which has no use for this new-fangled departure from classical specificity theory. Among other critics, Crue and Carregal first explain that they do not regard pain as a primary sensory modality, and that pain is not really even a sensation but is largely an emotionally charged 'percept'. They then proceed to criticize Wall, Melzack and Casey, proponents of gate control theory, because, they allege, 'they basically still consider pain as a sensation and are conceptualizing the presynaptic . . . modulation of a pattern of more or less specific excitatory or inhibitory peripheral balanced input. It is just not enough.'[36] Such criticisms testify to the fertility of gate control theory in promoting new research and theorizing in a rapidly expanding field of endeavour.

The Implications of the Theories

The adequacy of the alternative theories may be assessed by testing their explanatory power in relation to the paradoxical conditions of pain which have been described. It is obvious that specificity theory is hardly adequate to account for the facts of phantom limb pain, causalgia or the neuralgic conditions that have been described. In these conditions the chief anomaly is the experience of massive pain when no stimuli, or very gentle stimuli, are being applied to the place where the pain is felt. It used to be argued in terms of specificity theory that, in the case of phantom limb pain, the pain was being generated from the stump of the limb. Sensations carried by the nerves of the stump may undoubtedly be involved, but that does not account for the fact that *a past pain* may continue to be reproduced in the phantom, unless one is prepared to believe that the stump itself carries the complex patterning of a memory. With causalgia the pain appears to be due to a *lack* of adequate stimuli, because the nerve supply from beyond the injury is partially cut off. Pattern theory or gate control theory (the latter being really an elaboration of the former) can account for this feature of causalgic pain very adequately, for there is evidence that the nerve fibres of small diameter begin to regenerate before the fibres of large diameter, and thus the pattern of stimuli received is unbalanced, and though gentle it will be perceived as pain. Similarly, with post-herpetic neuralgia and the *tic douloureux*, the trouble arises from selective destruction of nerve fibres; hence the unbalanced pattern of stimuli received.

It must not be thought that the specificity theory of Von Frey was incorrect in terms of the knowledge available in his time. He made a valuable contribution in bringing forward evidence that there were a variety of sense receptors in the skin and elsewhere, and that they responded to a specific range of stimuli. However, it later became apparent that it was incorrect to label certain ranges and frequencies of neural firing 'pain'. All that the neurons convey is coded messages, some coming from the seat of the injury and some from within the sensorium itself, which have to be integrated and synthesized before the experience of pain can be generated. Some identical components of these coded messages can be synthesized with other neural messages and either cancelled or synthesized into 'pleasure'. An example of the latter phenomenon is Pavlov's well-known experiment[37] which involved teaching a dog to salivate in pleasurable expectancy of a food reward when given the signal of a mild electric shock on a certain site on its leg. The strength of the shock was gradually increased over a number of days until it was eventually so powerful that it was burning the animal's skin; yet the dog still responded with pleasure. If the shock was applied to any other site on its body, the dog would yelp with pain. This experiment emphasizes the importance of conditioning and memory in the generation of pain and pleasure.

Another deficiency of specificity theory is its failure to account for the facts about the surgical remedies used for the treatment of conditions of paradoxical pain. Attempts to remedy such conditions by cutting through the nerve tracts that lie between the place where pain is experienced and the brain are often unsuccessful.[38] An operation has sometimes been performed on the brain itself, the surgeon cutting out a piece of neural tissue at the exact spot of the sensory cortex where the affected part of the body is represented. Such an operation may have catastrophic results, for according to Wyke:

> The one thing this system does not contribute to is the pain; it does not hurt through this system. You can do what you like surgically to this system in a patient in pain and it doesn't make any difference other than to produce an acute confusional state because now the

patient has a pain he cannot localize, which previously he was able to localize. A psychiatric disturbance may follow when a patient 'has a pain' but does not know where it is. This is what happened in the early days when surgeons thought that this was all there was to the system, and they used to cut out bits of this system, for technically it is a very simple procedure, only to produce states of confusion and extreme distress and profound depression, and a number of their patients committed suicide.[39]

The difference between theories of patterning and summation on the one hand, and gate control theory on the other, is that in addition to the exactly specified mechanism of the spinal gate, the latter theory gives considerably more emphasis to the role of the brain and the psychological condition of the individual in determining what stimuli shall be admitted to the higher centres, and how they will be interpreted. It is this feature of gate control theory which has commended it to many modern research workers who study pain, whether or not they agree with the exact mechanisms proposed. Naturally, of the two authors of the theory it is the psychologist, Melzack, who has stressed the psychological aspects, and the neurophysiologist, Wall, the physiological.

In conclusion, it should be pointed out that all the conditions of paradoxical pain that have been described are precipitated or aggravated not only by physical stimuli but by psychological upsets. Pilowsky and Kaufman[40] cite the case of a man whose pains in a phantom limb were precipitated by witnessing or ruminating about scenes of violence. Similarly, causalgic attacks may be precipitated by emotional excitement, as described by Webb and Davis.[41] Psychological therapy in its various forms such as hypnosis,[42] distraction conditioning[43] and placebo treatment[44] can be of great benefit in treating cases of paradoxical pain where other methods have failed.

Towards a Definition of Pain

So much has been written about pain it might be thought that it would be easy to define just what is meant by the word. In fact this is not the case. The difficulty is not so much that different authorities give different definitions, but that they generally agree that although we all know what we mean by pain it is the sort of concept that defies definition. Merskey and Spear write:

Pain is one of these words whose use we understand very well, but which is difficult to define in a few words. . . . This difficulty has baffled many distinguished authors including Lewis (1942), Livingston (1943), Medvei (1949), Holmes (1950), Kolb (1954), Adrian (1956), Bishop (1956), Lhermitte (1957) and Beecher (1959), all of whom held it is difficult, or impossible to define the concept of pain.[45]

Other writers acknowledge the problem, but, feeling that it is incumbent on them to make an attempt, commit themselves to a rather rambling discourse. For example, Sternbach has written:

It is certainly not satisfying to look into the several ramifications and implications of our attempts to define pain, and to come away with the conclusion that no single definition is possible. We feel a lack of closure. It is then tempting to say 'Everyone knows what pain is anyway, so let's get on with the rest of the discussion'. But we cannot accept an assertion that implies that all of us share a common understanding of the matter, and so we will try two things. One is to attempt a definition, and the other is to be clear in the subsequent chapters, about what aspect of the definition we are dealing with.[46]

Later in his book Sternbach gives his definition:

Pain is the total set of responses an individual makes to a stimulus which causes or is about to cause tissue damage. These responses may be described in neurological, physiological, behavioural or affective terms.[47]

This is indeed a strange sort of definition, and seems to be an attempt to attempt definition in terms of naïve behaviourism. What Sternbach is defining is not *pain* but *pain behaviour*, and here he falls into the trap noted by Wyke, and quoted earlier, that the various concomitants of pain are simply epiphenomena. Indeed, such epiphenomena are not unique to pain: gasping, grimacing, crying out, a bounding pulse and raised blood pressure may equally be signs of acute pleasure, as every ardent lover knows. The only behavioural difference between the states of acute pain and pleasure, is that in the former the animal seeks to escape from it, and in the latter the animal seeks to prolong it. Even here the difference is not absolutely clear, for in some cases of, say, a sexual encounter, one partner may appear to be struggling free, but with squeals of delight.

Many modern writers agree that pain can be defined only in an ostensive manner, that is, by giving many examples in which the use of the term is appropriate. Indeed, it is difficult for an adult to remember a time when, as a child, he did not fully understand the meaning of the word 'pain', as children soon learn by ostensive definitions. Hilgard and Hilgard write:

> There is a triad of distress, incompletely described by sense perception, that includes *sensory pain, suffering*, and *mental anguish*. These concepts are familiar to lawyers who become engaged in controversies over personal injuries. It is no wonder that problems of definition arise.[48]

The Hilgards' reference to a 'triad of distress' is used by some writers, but in general it is the two-fold aspect of pain that is described, the *sensory component* and the *suffering*. One drastic remedy for chronic pain is the surgical operation of orbito-frontal leucotomy, whereby the fibres that go up from the thalamus to this part of the frontal cortex are transected. The result is that the patient is still aware of sensory stimuli coming up from the affected part of his body, but the suffering component is largely removed, so that he is no longer 'in pain'.[49] Alternatively, the operation may be carried out on the thalamus itself, which may be a safer procedure in some cases.[50]

Such brain surgery always has certain hazards, so it is rightly regarded as a last resort, and the cases in which it is likely to be successful require very careful selection. As a quote from Wyke earlier in this chapter made clear, in past times surgeons made the mistake of removing the *sensory* component of pain by ablating an area of the sensory cortex where the painful part of the body was represented, but the patient's *suffering* remained. One is reminded of a passage from *Hard Times* by Charles Dickens, that acute observer of human behaviour, in which an old lady lies dying:

> 'I think there's a pain somewhere in the room,' said Mrs Gradgrind, 'but I couldn't positively say that I have got it'.[51]

The dying lady has lost the sense of location of her pain.

If, therefore, we accept that pain normally consists of a combination of suffering and a sensory component, there are two alternative ways of looking at it. The first is to conceive of neural impulses arriving in the brain to signify pain, at which moment the person experiences suffering. This was the view of Wolff and Wolf,[52] who regarded the suffering as a 'reaction component'; these authors wrote from the viewpoint of the specificity theory, regarding pain as a sensation. An alternative, and more modern, view conceptualizes neural impulses arriving at different parts of the brain, each contributing simultaneously to the complex experience of pain. The concept of 'suffering' is itself complex, and is sometimes referred to as the 'motivational-affective' component of pain, for the essential feature which may be observed either by introspection, listening to verbal descriptions, or observing the behaviour of sufferers, is the emotional upset which drives us to 'do something about' the condition. Here it is significant that the most frontal part of the cortex is associated with motivation. Prefrontal leucotomy used to be used extensively with psychiatric patients whose lives were rendered unbearable by chronic worry.

At this point in our attempt to establish an adequate ostensive definition of pain we encounter the difficult question of distinguishing between pain and anxiety. We all know what it is like to have one without the other, although the extremes of anxiety generally have strong and most unpleasant pains associated with them. According to the old James-Lange theory of emotions, the physical awareness *is* the emotion, and the theory is expressed in such paradoxical statements as 'We feel sorry because we cry, and angry because we strike'.[53] This controversial view was at one time the subject of much inquiry by investigators such as Cannon and Sherrington, but it is no longer seriously entertained. The general view now is that emotions and their physiological and behavioural expressions can be considered as separate entities, although the emotion can be meaningfully discussed in terms of electro-chemical processes in the brain.

If, therefore, we are prepared to accept the general view that pain and anxiety (or 'physical pain' and 'mental pain') are separate entities, we can then proceed to examine the relationship between them.

REFERENCES

1 See W. Penfield and T. Rasmussen, *The Cerebral Cortex of Man*, New York: Macmillan, 1950.

2 R. Melzack, *The Puzzle of Pain*, Harmondsworth: Penguin Books, 1973, p. 76.

3 J. Hughes, 'Isolation of an endogenous compound from the brain with pharmacological properties similar to morphine', *Brain Research*, 1975, 88, pp. 295–308. See also J. W. Hughes and H. W. Kosterlitz, 'Opioid peptides', *British Medical Bulletin*, 1977, 33, p. 157.

4 For a useful discussion of older theories see K. M. Dallenbach, 'Pain: History and present status', *American Journal of Psychology*, 1939, 52, pp. 331–47.

5 St Thomas Aquinas, *Summa Theologiae*, 1a-2ae, XI, 1 ad 3.

6 B. Spinoza, *Ethics*, Part 3, Prop. II.

7 R. Descartes, *Treatise of Man*, (Trans. T. S. Hall), Cambridge, Mass: Harvard University Press, 1972.

8 See J. Breuer and S. Freud, 'Studies on hysteria', in J. Strachey (ed.), *Complete Works of Sigmund Freud*, Vol. 2, London: Hogarth Press, 1955, p. 178.

9   T. Szasz, 'A psychiatric perspective on pain and its control', op. cit.

10 B. D. Wyke, 'Neurological mechanisms in pain', Lecture at Middlesex Hospital Medical School, 12 November, 1972.

11 See M. L. Simmel, 'On phantom limbs', *Archives of Neurology and Psychiatry*, 1956, 75, pp. 637–47.

12 See B. Feinstein, J. C. Luce and J. N. K. Langton, 'The incidence of phantom limbs', in P. Klopsteg and P. Wilson (eds), *Human Limbs and Their Substitutes*, New York: McGraw-Hill, 1954.

13 See S. Sunderland, *Nerves and Nerve Injuries*, Edinburgh: E. & S. Livingstone, 1968.

14 H. Cohen, 'The mechanism of visceral pain,' *Transactions of the Medical Society of London*, 1944, 64, pp. 65–74.

15 L. C. Kolb, *The Painful Phantom: Psychology, Physiology and Treatment*, Springfield, Ill.: C. C. Thomas, 1954.

16 T. S. Szasz, *Pain and Pleasure: A Study of Bodily Feelings*, London: Tavistock Publications, 1957.

17 M. L. Simmel, 'Phantoms, phantom pain and "denial"', *American Journal of Psychotherapy*, 1959, 13, pp. 603–13.

18 J. R. Ewalt, G. C. Randall and H. Morris, 'The phantom limb', *Psychosomatic Medicine*, 1947, 9, pp. 118–23.

19 See R. Melzack, *The Puzzle of Pain*, op. cit., p. 56.

20 S. Weir Mitchell, *Injuries of Nerves and Their Consequences*, London: Smith, Elder & Co., 1872.

21 W. Noordenbos, *Pain*, Amsterdam: Elsevier Press, 1959.

22 Idem, 'An experimental approach to pain', in A. Soulairac, J. Cahn and J. Charpentier (eds), *Pain*, London: Academic Press, 1968.

23 See F. W. L. Kerr and R. H. Miller, 'The pathology of trigeminal neuralgia', *Archives of Neurology*, 1966, 15, pp. 308–19.

24 C. S. Sherrington, *The Integrative Actions of the Central Nervous System*, London: Constable, 1906.

25 A. Goldscheider, *'Ueber den Schmerz in physiologischer und klinischer Hinsicht*, Berlin: Hirschwald, 1894.

26 G. Weddell, 'Somesthesia and the chemical senses', *Annual Review of Psychology*, 1955, 6, pp. 119–36.

27 W. K. Livingston, *Pain Mechanisms*, New York: Macmillan, 1943.

28 G. H. Bishop, 'The relations between fibre size and sensory modality: philogenetic implications of the afferent innervation of the cortex', *Journal of Nervous and Mental Disease*, 1959, 128, pp. 89–114.

29 W. Noordenbos, *Pain*, op. cit.

30 R. Melzack and P. D. Wall, 'Pain mechanisms: A new theory', op. cit.

31 P. D. Wall, 'Modulation of pain by non-painful events', in J. J. Bonica and D. Albe-Fessard (eds), *Advances in Pain Research and Therapy*, New York: Raven Press, 1976.

32 R. Melzack and P. D. Wall, 'Pain mechanisms: A new theory', op. cit.

33 R. F. Schmidt, 'The gate control theory of pain: An unlikely hypothesis', in J. P. Payne and R. A. P. Burt (eds), *Pain,* London: Churchill Livingstone, 1972.

34 P. D. Wall, 'Modulation of pain by non-painful events', op. cit.

35 V. B. Mountcastle, *Medical Physiology*, 13th Edition, St Louis: C. V. Mosby, 1974.

36 B. L. Crue and E. J. A. Carregal, 'Postsynaptic repetitive neuron discharge in

neuralgic pain', in J. J. Bonica (ed.), *Advances in Neurology*, Vol 4, New York: Raven Press, 1974, p. 645.

37 See I. Pavlov, *Conditioned Reflexes*, New York: Oxford University Press, 1927.

38 See S. Sunderland, *Nerves and Nerve Injuries*, op. cit.

39 B. D. Wyke, 'Neurological mechanisms in pain', op. cit.

40 I. Pilowsky and A. Kaufman, 'An experimental study of atypical phantom pain', *British Journal of Psychiatry*, 1965, 111, pp. 1185-7.

41 E. M. Webb and E. W. Davis, 'Causalgia: A review', *Californian Medicine*, 1948, 69, pp. 412-7.

42 See C. Cedercreutz and E. Uusitalo, 'Hypnotic treatment of phantom sensations in 37 amputees', in J. Lassner (ed.), *Hypnosis in Psychosomatic Medicine*, New York: Springer-Verlag, 1967.

43 See F. S. Morgenstern, 'The effects of sensory input and concentration on post-amputation phantom limb pain', *Journal of Neurology, Neurosurgery and Psychiatry*, 1964, 27, pp. 55-65.

44 See R. A. Sternbach, *Pain: A Psychophysiological Analysis*, New York: Academic Press, 1968.

45 H. Merskey and F. G. Spear, *Pain: Psychological and Psychiatric Aspects*, op. cit., p. 14.

46 R. A. Sternbach, *Pain Patients*, op. cit., p. 11.

47 Ibid., p. 159.

48 E. R. Hilgard and J. R. Hilgard, *Hypnosis in the Relief of Pain*, Los Altos, Calif.: W. Kaufmann, 1975, p. 29.

49 See W. Freeman and J. W. Watts, *Psychosurgery in the Treatment of Mental Disorders and Intractable Pain*, Springfield, Ill.: C. C. Thomas, 1950.

50 See V. H. Mark, F. R. Ervin and P. I. Yakolev, 'Stereotactic thalamotomy', *Archives of Neurology*, 1963, 8, pp. 528-38.

51 C. Dickens, *Hard Times*, (Household Edition), London: Chapman & Hall, 1877, p. 80.

52 H. G. Wolff and S. Wolf, *Pain*, 2nd Edition, Springfield, Ill.: C. C. Thomas, 1958.

53 See W. James, *Psychology: Briefer Course*, London: Macmillan, 1892.

4

EMOTIONS AND THE PERCEPTUAL
APPROACH TO PAIN

In the preceding chapter an attempt was made to discuss theories of pain and to arrive at some definition of its nature. The present chapter will discuss the relationship of the emotions of rage, fear and anxiety to pain, and to present evidence for the view that pain can most usefully be regarded in terms of the psychology of perception.

It is widely recognized that if we are acutely anxious, we are prone to experience as painful physical events which would not normally cause pain. Furthermore, a mildly painful condition such as moderate post-surgical trauma will be greatly magnified if any circumstance raises the anxiety level of the patient. The placebo treatment of conditions of pain relates to this relationship between anxiety and pain, and some writers such as Barber[1] hold that hypnosis acts to reduce or abolish pain simply through an anxiety-reducing mechanism, a view which is not wholly supported by the experimental evidence, as shown by Orne.[2]

The relationship between anxiety and pain is complex. To take the case of a patient undergoing surgery, the anticipation of the operation will naturally raise his anxiety level and hence his proneness to experience a higher level of pain than the physical procedure justifies. Interesting research has been carried out with patients awaiting operations. Egbert and his associates found that the drug pentobarbitol, which is frequently given to calm patients in the pre-operative period, was not so effective in reducing post-operative pain as a simple visit and reassuring chat by the anaesthetist.[3] In a further study Egbert's team found that the reduction of anxiety achieved by this visit secured a reduction of 50 per cent in the post-operative narcotics required, and that the visited patients were ready for discharge from hospital an average of 2.7 days earlier than a control group who had not been visited.[4] The association between anxiety and the degree of pain which surgical patients will suffer is now well recognized, and in enlightened hospitals it is standard practice for the patient to be visited for ten minutes or so by an anaesthetist before his operation.

In 1959 Beecher[5] published some studies of battle casualties and of injured civilians which shed considerable light on the relationship between anxiety and pain, but which raised an interesting paradox. It was observed that among severely wounded soldiers treated at casualty stations only one out of three complained of pain to the degree that they required morphine. These wounded men were not numb, for they could clearly feel and resent a clumsy needle jab, but their severe wounds did not appear to cause them as much pain as the doctors, who had experience of wounds in civil life, expected. The paradox is: if, as one would expect, the conditions of battle naturally create high anxiety, why did these wounded soldiers experience little pain compared with civilians in similar circumstances?

After the war, Beecher returned to civilian practice, and studied the pain responses of people injured in accidents. He observed that people who had sustained injuries comparable to those of the soldiers appeared to suffer a great deal more pain. He has suggested that an essential difference was to be found in the meaning of the wound for the individual: for the soldier a wound meant an honourable escape from the threat of death on the battlefield, but for the injured civilian his accident was generally a calamity.

This is probably not an adequate explanation for the difference, for although escape from the battlefield brings relief, the battle wounds were sustained in a situation highly productive of emotion, and realizing that one is mutilated has its own problems. Perhaps part of the difference lies in the distinction which must be made between 'rage', 'fear' and 'anxiety'. On the battlefield the soldiers may be said to be in a condition of 'rage' and 'fear'; 'rage' may also apply to some athletes in competitive sports where a marked insensitivity to pain is observed. By contrast, civilians who are the victims of a sudden accident are in no sense emotionally prepared, and what they afterwards suffer is more a matter of 'anxiety'. It is not an either/or distinction, for several conditions may co-exist to some degree in an animal.[6] As well as there being behavioural differences which cause us to attach different labels to recognizable patterns of animal responses, there are also different physiological concomitants of these states. In states of fear there is an increase of the hormone adrenalin in the system; in states of rage, in addition to increased adrenalin there is also an increase in nor-adrenalin. Both hormones produce changes in the viscera, muscular tone and glandular secretions which adapt the body for emergency action, but there are slight differences which relate to whether the dominant pattern of action shall be flight or fighting. Experimental studies with man and other animals upon which this theory rests have been reviewed by Kopin.[7] What has not yet been fully clarified experimentally, although it is a plausible hypothesis, is whether the neurophysiological changes associated with rage and fear are significantly related to the secretion of endorphins, the body's own pain-killing chemicals, in human beings.

The PDR Model of Fear and Pain

A most interesting paper has recently been published by Bolles and Fanselow[8] on what they call the 'perceptual-defensive-recuperative' (PDR) theoretical model. This is largely based on experimental work with animals, and discusses a new theory about fear and pain. They suggest that in conditions of fear the body secretes endorphins, thus rendering the frightened animal relatively immune to pain. Such relative immunity would mean that efforts made to escape or to repel an attacker would not be inhibited by pain attendant on any wounds it received. These authors provide a novel theory of fear and pain: the former they regard as an independent motivating system which organizes the body to its maximum efficiency not only for coping physically, but for perceiving the salient features of the emergency situation, e.g. in perceiving avenues of escape. This is a valuable point of view about fear because we may be too apt (drawing on human experience) to over-stress its disorganizing effects.

Bolles and Fanselow's view of pain is rather more novel: they regard it as an independent motivating system, the purpose of which is to make the wounded animal withdraw quietly and engage in recuperative behaviour. Here they cite a paper by Wall[9] in which this idea is discussed, suggesting that the wounded deer may be immune to pain whilst it is frightened, and hence will run and engage in other defensive behaviour, unhampered by pain, until it is in a safe place, when it will become aware of the smart of its wounds and will be dominated by recuperative behaviour.

This PDR theoretical model envisages behaviour being controlled by independent and antagonistic motivational systems. However, in postulating that fear inhibits pain, the model would demand that pain inhibits fear. Ordinary experience would suggest that the latter is not the case; many of us may remember being frightened whilst we were in pain. Bolles and Fanselow answer this objection as follows:

A particularly interesting question is whether pain inhibits fear. . . . The different motivational systems occur in a sort of natural hierarchy, with some motives taking priority over others. Because of the urgency with which the need for defensive behaviour may arise, fear should have top priority, easily inhibiting other systems, but itself being difficult to inhibit. Pain has less urgency and so should have a lower priority.[10]

The idea that fear inhibits pain is indeed plausible, whether or not all the experimental evidence that these authors cite, attributing the inhibition of pain to the agency of endorphins, is acceptable. It would certainly explain the case of soldiers on the battlefield feeling relatively less pain from their wounds than might be expected, and also the well-known phenomenon of the person who is abnormally frightened of dental treatment finding that his toothache suddenly disappears when he arrives in the dentist's waiting-room. Nevertheless, Bolles and Fanselow have to admit to an anomaly in their theory, an anomaly that is met with in the clinical situation. They write:

> Fear, which usually competes with and effectively inhibits pain, appears under certain circumstances to have the contrary effect of sensitizing an individual to pain. Clinically, one of the problems of dealing with pain is the management of fear that may be caused by the pain (the patient may not be able to cope with it) or by worrying about the cause of pain (the patient may think he is dying). Once these fears are allayed, the original pain may be much easier to treat or may even disappear spontaneously.[11]

They cite the example of childbirth in which the woman's unnecessary pain may be reduced by appropriate training which removes her fear of the event. They also acknowledge that drugs such as alcohol which reduce fear, also reduce pain. It seems that these instances directly contradict the thesis that they are trying to establish, and they go on to write:

> The practical principle here is quite clear: deal with the fear first, and then pain will be a minor problem. But the explanation of the principle is elusive. Why should fear increase pain? Fear is hypothesized to activate the endorphins; it should reduce the pain induced by noxious stimulation. How can it sensitize the pain system?[12]

Their answer to this question is twofold: first they cite the fairly well-known theory that as a state of fear may produce muscle tension, conditions such as headache are supposed to be brought on by tensions in the muscles of the head and neck. This is not a very satisfactory explanatory theory, and quite appropriately they ask, 'Where is the tooth muscle that is tense when I worry that the dentist will make my tooth hurt?'

Their solution to this puzzle is a very curious one. They suggest that it is not really pain from which the frightened patient suffers, but his fear. They conceive of the patient mis-labelling his condition of distress: because he knows that he has been 'hurt', he thinks of himself as being 'in pain'. This very novel view derives from their conception of pain as a motivational state of recuperation, and fear as a motivational state of self-defence. The patient, writhing in what he regards as pain, is in a state of active self-defence; *ergo* he is not in pain but in fear!

The journal *The Behavioral and Brain Sciences*, in which this article was published, is one which publishes the comments of critics in the same issue, and the Bolles and Fanselow article is followed by twenty-one short critical commentaries. The original article is long and deals with a great deal of technical matter concerning conditioning theory which will not be discussed here. One of the critics, Greenberg,[13] makes a point which should be appreciated by the layman, that our knowledge about endorphins, which have only recently been discovered, is as yet scanty and that we should still be cautious in invoking them as an explanatory factor in theorizing about pain. Also, as Fonberg[14] points out, we do not know definitely whether or not fear can induce the release of endorphins independently of pain. Fields[15] states that 'Our own observations and those of others suggest that pain alone may activate the endorphin-mediated analgesia system.'

Perhaps the most contentious aspect of PDR theory, as set out in the article, is the novel suggestion referred to above that the writhing patient is not in a state of pain but of fear. A number of commentators comment on the semantics of this argument. Vierck and Cooper remark:

> It seems to us that both pain and fear can elicit defensive or recuperative behaviours; and they can both elicit similar emotional states, motivational vectors, perceptual experiences, and levels and patterns of autonomic and somatic activity. Both the clinical and the laboratory animal literatures indicate that the emotional behaviours and feelings accompanying pain can range over the gamut of supposedly negative and positive affect states, including agony, sexual arousal, depression, laughter, fear, rage, aggression, and submission.[16]

A fact that none of the commentators mention, and which may indeed be significant, is that as Bolles and Fanselow are psychologists who have worked chiefly with rats, this may have influenced their view of emotional behaviour and experience. The rat, although a very convenient laboratory animal, is relatively low on the phylogenetic scale, and does not share the complex psychology of the higher mammals, including man. Some thirty years ago there was a great deal of experimentation with the higher mammals by researchers such as Masserman,[17] attempting to induce 'experimental neuroses', that is, states which may be comparable with the anxiety states which are suffered by human beings. Later researchers such as Broadhurst[18] attempted to repeat this work with rats, but it was found that while rats could certainly experience fear, and indeed there were rats with greater and lesser degrees of emotionality, the rat is too simple an animal to experience anything that might reasonably be called 'anxiety', if we use the term as it relates to the human species. It seems meaningful to use 'fear' in Bolles and Fanselow's sense to refer to an immediate alarm reaction to threatened or actual harm, which may very well result in the system being flooded with pain-killing endorphins, but anxiety is another matter. Using introspection, we may say that anxiety is often not concerned with any very immediate threat, but is a long-term brooding over possible dangers; it is typical of the human species with its well developed concern for the future, typified by its enlarged frontal lobes of the brain. All the clinical evidence indicates that it is anxiety rather than fear which exacerbates pain, and that individuals who are more prone to anxiety are least able to tolerate pain. If we accept the essential difference between anxiety and fear, then there are no contradictions which have to be met by semantic gymnastics.

Another feature of Bolles and Fanselow's article is that they do not consider the emotion of rage, which is specially productive of analgesia, possibly through the agency of endorphins. In commenting on their article, Eysenck remarks:

It seems likely that any strong motivational state will inhibit the perception of pain, so that fear is only one of a number of different motivational states having the same effect. As any sportsman knows, painful injury suffered during a game, or some competition in which the person involved is very actively engaged at a high level of motivation, is hardly felt at all until the end of the game or competition; these occasions do not involve fear in any way.[19]

Whether their omission of any reference to rage is also due to a preoccupation with rats, which are studied mostly at the receiving end of noxious stimuli, is difficult to determine. Studies of other species (including humans) in conditions of active aggression when there is little component of fear, may reveal that when we put on our war-paint we also equip ourselves with a liberal dose of endorphins, so that pain does not inhibit our aggressive behaviour.

Bolles and Fanselow's article, which has been discussed at some length, is of interest as it is indicative of an important direction of pain research in the 1980s in experimental laboratories of psychology and the neurosciences. This new departure from the old approach of treating the body as though it were 'hard-wired' for pain has developed from the new conception of pain as a perceptual phenomenon, and from a body of research which has drawn very widely on different scientific disciplines.

Pain Regarded as a Percept

If we regard pain as a percept, then it follows that it can be measured, understood, and indeed controlled by the methods that have been developed in the study of perceptual phenomena. The term 'perception' is technical: it refers to the process whereby raw sense data are organized by the higher centres of the brain and rendered meaningful. That such an elaborating process is entirely necessary before we can make any sense of the world about us is not perhaps immediately apparent, but the following example will illustrate the essential difference between receiving sensory information and building it into a meaningful percept. Senden[20] studied patients who were born blind because of the opacity of the cornea of their eyes, but when the operation for cataract became possible they were given perfectly normal eyes in adulthood. At first they could make very little sense of what they saw; for instance, they could not readily distinguish between a triangle and a rectangle, having to count the corners. It took several weeks of sight experience before these patients could learn to build up meaningful percepts from the jumble of patterns presented to the retina of their eyes, and conveyed in neural signals to the visual cortex. To some degree this natural experiment can be compared with that of Melzack and Scott[21] who reared puppies in an artificially padded and pain-free environment. When grown-up, these dogs could not perceive pain in a normal manner, but would repeatedly make maladaptive actions, such as putting their noses into flames. It is well established that perception of our environment involves a process of learning.

All perceptual phenomena are entirely private experiences: I can only know that a man hears a distant cuckoo, or smells roses, or sees a detail in a picture, or feels pain, because he tells me so. When the sense data are very faint he may indeed be mistaken as to the veridicality of his perceptions – he may claim to smell roses when there are no such flowers around. Special techniques such as hypnotic suggestion may cause such non-veridical percepts to be experienced. The percept of pain is in a rather special category since it refers to events wholly within the nervous system without any external object to which they refer. If a person claims to experience pain it is nonsense to to say that he is 'mistaken' because there is no readily detectable reason why he should have that experience.

The study of pain in a relatively new body of research, that of Sensory Decision Theory (SDT), is a very promising approach and illustrates many of the points made in the last chapter. SDT has not entirely replaced the older methods of studying perceptual experience, known as *pychophysics*, but exists as a distinct outgrowth from it. Psychophysics is basically the study of the relation of the energy of a stimulus to the reported intensity of the sensation it produces. It began in the mid nineteenth century and is associated with the name of the philosopher and scientist Fechner; later it was used by Von Frey in 1894 in an attempt to measure human pain. A review of this classical work and its later developments is given by Wolff.[22]

Suppose we try to detect a very faint stimulus against a background of noise, say the occasional sound of a distant ship's siren against the constant boom of the sea; sometimes we are sure we hear it; sometimes we wonder if it is our imagination. What we are concerned with is the signal to noise ratio, and this can be demonstrated to have interesting properties which relate to the psychological state of the *observer* (the person who hears, sees or otherwise experiences a stimulus). In laboratory experiments the observer is presented with a constant background of 'noise' (the term 'noise' is used to refer to any modality and not necessarily hearing) and occasionally presented with a stimulus, at first at a very weak intensity, without warning; he is required to detect when it is 'present' and 'absent'. As the stimulus is so faint the observer is encouraged to guess, i.e. to make a decision on the basis of very slight evidence, and the results of a repeated number of trials are recorded in a table such as that shown below.

Judgements

	'absent'	'present'
Stimulus given	a	b (HR)
Stimulus not given	c	d (FAR)

When judgements are in cells b or c they are veridical (i.e. in accord with objective reality), but cells a and d represent two types of errors of judgement. Type a error consists of failing to detect a stimulus which is present because of the masking 'noise'; type d error consists of mistaking some of the 'noise' for the stimulus. This is not just a matter of sensory physiology; it depends upon the psychological 'set' of the observer, which may be related to some aspects of his basic personality. A cautious person will, in a laboratory setting, make many type a errors; a rash or highly imaginative person will tend to make type d errors. Obviously the greater the background of 'noise' the more difficult the task of detection will be, and the stimulus must be of greater intensity before it can be detected.

We must remember that in real life a stimulus *never* comes to our brain alone; what is perceived is always 'noise'-plus-stimulus, for the nervous system is never inactive. We are constantly being bombarded with stimuli, generated both externally and internally, and isolation experiments have shown that we become very distressed if the level of bombardment is substantially reduced over a period of time.

Cell b in the table is labelled HR (hit rate) and cell d FAR (false affirmative rate). By relating HR to FAR in the results given by any individual, we can establish two pieces of information about his performance; (i) his perceptual sensitivity, and (ii) the bias of his responses due to his personal style of making decisions. Sensory sensitivity, sometimes given the symbol d', represents the ability of an individual to detect the difference between 'noise'-plus-stimulus and 'noise' alone. Indeed, as the stimuli which are too weak will *never* be detected, d' can represent the ability to detect the difference between 'noise'-plus-stimulus X and 'noise'-plus-stimulus Y, where X and Y represent different intensities.

A positive response bias represents a 'set' to maximize the HR; a negative bias represents an attempt to minimize the FAR. As pointed out above, the direction and strength of this bias represents both transient situational factors, and factors relating to enduring personality traits. In a situation involving pain, when a local anaesthetic has been applied, naturally d' is reduced, and the recipient of possibly painful stimuli, *knowing* that his skin has been anaesthetized, will change the bias of his judgements as to how strong stimuli have to be before he will label them as being 'painful'. If instead of applying a real local anaesthetic to his skin we apply a neutral lotion, but solemnly assure him that it is an anaesthetic, this placebo is also likely to change the bias of his judgements. Not only will he report less pain but he will actually feel less pain. This may be difficult to believe, but it is true beyond all doubt that placebos have the power of altering the psychological state to the extent that the experience of pain is substantially reduced. This applies not only to minor pains inflicted in a laboratory, but to the severe pain encountered in hospital wards. Paradoxically, it is in the latter setting that placebos are the most effective. Placebos work much more effectively with some people than with others. Why this should be so, remains a mystery; the relevant differences in personality have not yet been established.[23]

An example from the 'real world' illustrates how SDT applies to the experience of small intensities of pain. If we have a slight nagging pain, say from a minor burn, we may not notice it at all during the day when the 'noise' level in the system is high due to our many activities, but when we are resting in the silent night and the level of 'noise' is low we may become conscious of this throbbing burn and experience it as painful.

Fechner's psychophysics was a stimulus-response (S-R) theory, anticipating Pavlov's later use of the concept. Thus, a given sensory stimulus (S) might be expected to produce an appropriate response (R), in terms of the sensation experienced. The later theory, SDT (which also stands for Signal Detection Theory), is sometimes written as S-O-R, the intermediate O standing for 'observer'; for whether a stimulus produces a response or not depends upon the psychological state of the observer. Whether an observer decides that he is experiencing a stimulus (i.e. is conscious of it) depends on all sorts of factors – how he interprets the present situation, the meaning the stimulus has for him, his past learning experience, his present beliefs and his basic personality. In Chapter 6 individual susceptibility to pain will be discussed, and the immense importance of the O in S-O-R will become apparent.

In the experimental context, or in real life, pain is a phenomenon uniquely different from experience in the sensory modalities of sight, hearing, touch, etc. If we are experimenting with, say, light, we can cut out the background 'noise' almost entirely by working in darkness, although even in the dark we appear to see self-generated flashes and patterns, just as when we close our eyes. We can however, make fairly definite discriminations between 'noise'-plus-stimulus and 'noise' alone, in the sense that it is not difficult to come to a decision whether the light is on or off. With pain the decision is much more difficult; it is not just a decision between 'pain' and 'no pain', for the background of 'noise' is so vast, and consists in fact of the totality of our sensory and indeed our emotional experience. The experience we sort out from the 'noise' background has to be categorized as 'pain', 'neutral feeling' or 'pleasure'. The decision process is very complex. An old theory held that pain was an experience in *any* modality of an unpleasantly great degree of intensity. While this simple theory is hardly tenable, it serves to remind us that pain and pleasure are qualities of experience that can enter into any sense modality.

The classic studies of the measurement of pain have typically involved several observations. First, the *threshold* – how intense a stimulus has to be before the recipient will decide that it is painful; second, the level of *toleration* – how intense the stimulus is when the recipient decides that it is unbearably painful, or alternatively, how long he will consent to bear a stimulus of constant strong intensity. The SDT work has introduced the new measure of d', a measure of sensory sensitivity, that throws doubt on the older idea that we could ever measure an absolute threshold, since it depends on fluctuating psychological processes. And finally there is the measure of *response bias*.

An interesting example of SDT in experimental work is that of Chapman *et al.*,[24] who investigated the effects of nitrous oxide. It is well known that this gas can produce total anaesthesia, but they wished to investigate scientifically its power in small doses to reduce sensitivity to pain. Comparing SDT measures of response to the pain generated by radiant heat, with volunteer human subjects, they found that the gas did two things; it reduced sensitivity to pain and it altered the response bias of the subjects so that they were less prone to report the stimulus as painful. It will be remembered that in 1844 Horace Wells the dentist noted that one of the young men, slightly intoxicated by the nitrous oxide provided by Gardner Colton at a lecture, severely damaged his shin but felt no pain. Going back to the beginning of the last century, we have noted how Coleridge and others claimed to experience positive pleasure from inhaling the gas. Here we have examples of sensory 'noise' in the system, despite being increased by a blow on the shin or by radiant heat, being either disregarded or processed to produce pleasure.

Diazepam is a drug which is not officially an analgesic; in its commercial form of Valium it is widely prescribed to reduce anxiety, but some clinicians report that it sometimes serves to reduce pain. Chapman and Feather[25] employed the pain engendered by a tourniquet to examine and compare the effects of diazepam, placebo and aspirin on the time that volunteer human subjects would tolerate the pain. They found that the length of time was increased by the use of diazepam, and as one might also expect, that the subjects reported being less anxious in the experiment whilst under the influence of the drug. In a second experiment with the same subjects these authors used radiant heat as a pain stimulus; analysing the results by the SDT method they found that diazepam had no effect on either sensitivity to pain or on response bias. These results suggest that any reduction in reaction to long-continued pain which diazepam produces is due to the motivational-emotional component of pain, and not to the perceptual experience of pain, as with nitrous oxide.

SDT has been used in various experiments designed to study placebo effects. Thus Clark[26] used SDT procedures in investigating how a placebo will increase response bias against reporting thermally-induced pain; he found that the placebo did not affect the subjects' sensitivity to changes in the intensity of the stimulus. This is rather a subtle point, and can perhaps best be expressed by saying that placebos do not 'dull' our sensitivity, but alter our subjective experience regarding what we are prepared to call pain. Similarly, Chapman and Butler[27] found that the antidepressant drug doxepin, and alternatively placebo pills, had the power strongly to affect the response bias in reporting pain from dental shocks given to healthy subjects, whilst leaving their sensitivity unaltered.

It is not proposed to give any adequate account of SDT here; Green and Swets[28] have explained the theory comprehensively and related it to the older body of psychophysics. Rollman[29] has recently criticized its applications to research into problems of pain, principally on the grounds that SDT is inappropriate for analysing conditions in which the pain stimulus is of high intensity, as in clinical studies of pain. Rollman maintains that in such conditions the measure d' reflects discrimination between different degrees of pain, but not pain sensitivity. Chapman[30] has answered this criticism, but it seems plain that, like the two housewives disputing across a street in Edinburgh whom Hume made famous, Rollman and he will never agree as they are arguing from different premises. Wolff has characterized SDT as having 'a kind of bandwagon effect on pain research, and many investigators consider that SDT is the only correct approach to psychophysical studies'.[31] Possibly it is a matter of those who investigate pain from a more psychological perspective finding that SDT is useful to them, whereas those who take a more physiological approach prefer the older form of psychophysics.

This area of research has been mentioned principally to emphasize the point of view taken in this book that the nature of pain can best be understood as a perceptual phenomenon existing against the perpetual background of 'noise' generated by the nervous system, rather than according to the 'push-button' concept of pain, originating with Descartes and elaborated by many of the nineteenth-century physiologists and their later followers. Only when one fully appreciates the essentially psychological nature of pain, does it become possible to understand the methods which are being developed in more recent times for the conquest of pain.

REFERENCES

1 T. X. Barber, *LSD, Marihuana, Yoga and Hypnosis*, op. cit.

2 M. T. Orne, 'Mechanisms of hypnotic pain control', in J. J. Bonica and D. Albe-Fessard (eds), *Advances in Pain Research and Therapy*, op. cit.

3 L. D. Egbert, G. E. Battit, H. Tundof and H. K. Beecher, 'The value of a pre-operative visit by an anaesthetist', *Journal of the American Medical Association*, 1963, 185, pp. 553-5.

4 L. D. Egbert, G. E. Battit, C. E. Welsh and M. K. Bartlett, 'Reduction of post-operative pain by encouragement and instruction of patients', *New England Journal of Medicine*, 1964, 270, pp. 825-7.

5 H. K. Beecher, *Measurement of Subjective Responses*, London: Oxford University Press, 1959.

6 See P. R. Marler and W. J. Hamilton, *Mechanisms of Animal Behavior*, New York: Wiley & Son, 1966.

7 I. J. Kopin, 'Catecholamines, adrenal hormones and stress', in D. T. Krieger and J. C. Hughes (eds), *Neuroendocrinology*, Sunderland, Mass.: Sinauer Associates, 1980.

8 R. C. Bolles and M. S. Fanselow, 'A perceptual-defensive-recuperative model of fear and pain', *The Behavioral and Brain Sciences*, 1980, 3, pp. 291–323.

9 P. D. Wall, 'On the relation of injury to pain', *Pain*, 1979, 6, pp. 253–64.

10 R. C. Bolles and M. S. Fanselow, op. cit., p. 299.

11 Ibid.

12 Ibid.

13 G. Greenberg, ibid., p. 310.

14 E. Fonberg, ibid., p. 309.

15 H. L. Fields, ibid., p. 308.

16 C. J. Vierck and B. J. Cooper, ibid., p. 314.

17 See J. H. Masserman, *Behaviour and Neurosis*, New York: Hefner, 1964.

18 See P. L. Broadhurst, 'Abnormal animal behaviour', in H. J. Eysenck (ed.), *Handbook of Abnormal Psychology*, London: Pitman, 1960.

19 H. J. Eysenck, in R. C. Bolles and M. S. Fanselow, op. cit. p. 308.

20 M. V. Senden, *Space and Sight*, (Trans. P. Heath), New York: Free Press, 1960.

21 R. Melzack and T. H. Scott, 'The effect of early experience on the response to pain', *Journal of Comparative and Physiological Psychology*, 1957, 50, pp. 155–61.

22 B. B. Wolff, 'Behavioural measurement of human pain', in R. A. Sternbach (ed.), *The Psychology of Pain*, New York: Raven Press, 1978.

23 See F. J. Evans, 'The placebo response in pain reduction', in J. J. Bonica (ed.), *Advances in Neurology*, op. cit.

24 C. R. Chapman, T. M. Murphy and S. H. Butler, 'Analgesic strength of 33 per cent nitrous oxide: A Signal Detection Theory evaluation', *Science*, 179, 1973, pp. 1246–8.

25 C. R. Chapman and B. W. Feather, 'Effects of diazepam on human pain tolerance and pain sensitivity', *Psychosomatic Medicine*, 1973, 35, pp. 330–40.

26 W. C. Clark, 'Sensory decision theory analysis of the placebo effect on the criterion for pain and thermal sensitivity', *Journal of Abnormal Psychology*, 1969, 73, pp. 363–71.

27 C. R. Chapman and S. H. Butler, 'Effects of doxepin on perception of laboratory induced pain in man', *Pain*, 1978, 5, pp. 253–62.

28 D. M. Green and J. A. Swets, *Signal Detection Theory and Psychophysics*, New York: R. E. Kruger Pub. Co., 1974.

29 G. B. Rollman, 'Signal Detection Theory measurement of pain: a review and critique', *Pain*, 1977, 3, pp. 187–211.

30 C. R. Chapman, 'Sensory Decision Theory methods in pain research: a reply to Rollman', *Pain*, 1977, 3, pp. 295–305.

31 B. B. Wolff, 'Behavioural measurement of human pain', op. cit., p. 143.

5

THE INHIBITION OF PAIN BY
HYPNOTIC SUGGESTION

Most people regard the abolition or attenuation of pain by hypnotic suggestion as a great mystery. The ambiguity of the topic is reflected in the extraordinary lack of interest shown in it by scientific circles through the centuries. This lack of interest still persists. At the First World Congress on Pain in 1975 numerous papers were presented by a wide variety of specialists in pain research, but of the 148 published papers only two were concerned with the inhibition of pain in humans by hypnosis.[1] This neglect is all the more remarkable in view of the steadily growing recognition of the importance of psychological techniques in the treatment of pain.

The reasons why the control of pain by hypnosis or by mesmerism (and the two are not the same thing) was vehemently opposed by medical and dental surgeons in the middle of the last century have been discussed in Chapter 2. The more conservative members of the medical profession originally opposed the use of all anaesthesia, but the more progressive doctors were struggling to get chemical anaesthesia accepted in spite of conservative opposition, and they did not wish to be associated with the foolish occultism that was professed by so many of the mesmerists. These reasons no longer apply today, for most scientists investigating and practising hypnosis have no use for the parapsychology which still lingers on the wilder shores of academe. That hypnosis continues to be cold-shouldered by most researchers into the control of pain is a problem which invites investigation.

The Nature of Hypnosis

Not least among the problems of considering hypnosis in the control of pain, is that there is no general agreement as to what precisely constitutes hypnosis. In discussing the nature of pain it was pointed out that it is extremely difficult to define pain, and that we must be content with an ostensive definition. It is even more difficult to define hypnosis,

91

and the ostensive definition of it must be even less precise. However, it is necessary that we should attempt some clarification in order that the mechanisms of hypnosis may be explained.

There are two main approaches to the conceptualization of hypnosis, which differ as to the extent that the phenomenon may be usefully conceptualized as an altered state of awareness. The 'state' theorists regard hypnosis in terms of a state of consciousness different from that of our ordinary waking state. The 'non-state' theorists prefer to regard hypnosis in terms of certain special interpersonal relationships. The 'state' theorists are in the direct scientific tradition of the Nancy School of the nineteenth century and its best-known writer Hyppolite Bernheim.[2] This school rejected the older formulations of the mesmerists who believed in the reality of 'animal magnetism': it taught that mesmeric and hypnotic phenomena were dependent on the capacities of the subject himself rather than the power of the hypnotist or mesmerist. Consequently, it emphasized the fact that individuals varied very much in their capacity, possibly innate, to enter an altered state of consciousness. This tradition is well represented today by the researchers at Stanford University and by the writings of Ernest Hilgard and his associates.[3] Other eminent 'state' theorists working elsewhere, such as Martin Orne, Kenneth Bowers and André Weitzenhoffer, have also made a distinguished contribution to the study of hypnosis.

'Non-state' theorists lay their emphasis not on the special personality characteristics of the subject which enable him, to a greater or lesser degree, to go into a trance state, but on *what is done to him*. They are more in the tradition of those who regarded the role of the operator (mesmerist or hypnotist) as crucial. Modern 'non-state' theorists do not, of course, believe in the reality of 'animal magnetism' or any such occult force: their general theoretical position is that the hypnotic subject acts as he does and has certain unusual experiences because of the very special social situation in which he finds himself, and it is not necessary to regard him as being in an altered state of consciousness. In this formulation, the hypnotist is of importance because he creates a social situation in which certain compelling interpersonal forces operate. Prominent among the 'non-state' theorists are Sarbin and Coe,[4] who have developed a theory of role-playing in which the hypnotized subject is regarded as enacting a very special role – that of 'being hypnotized' as he understands it, and as continuously defined by the hypnotist. It must not be thought that these theorists regard hypnosis as being in any way sham behaviour adopted to deceive and impress the hypnotist and any onlookers. They regard all role-playing as a perfectly genuine performance which is believed in by the performer.

Many people regard the special weakness of the role theorists' conception of hypnosis as being revealed in their attempts to explain hypnotic analgesia. The critics ask how a man under hypnosis can endure a severe surgical operation without pain simply by playing the role of an analgesic subject? Role-playing seems perhaps too glib an explanation. In criticizing the role theorists, Hilgard calls attention to the case cited by Sarbin and Coe of a patient who felt no pain when his wrist was burned while it was hypnotically anaesthetic. These authors stated that:

> The patient had to choose between disclosing that he felt the burn, thereby embarrassing and perhaps displeasing the therapist on whom he had become dependent, or not disclosing the private fact that he felt the burn and thus avoiding the risk of weakening the relationship.[5]

Hilgard comments that 'The implication that a person reports no pain only because he wishes to keep a secret from the hypnotherapist is a misleading exaggeration of social role theory.'[6] In this particular instance Sarbin and Coe are certainly slipping into a mode of explanation which involves the concept of a sort of mere shamming, but their general level of conceptualization is more sophisticated. The present author asked William Coe to explain in more detail exactly what was his attitude to the inhibition of pain by hypnotic suggestion, and received the following reply:

> I believe that your statement . . . 'still left puzzling as to how someone can *effectively* play the role of experiencing no pain when he is undergoing a severe surgical operation, etc.' – suggests that you have misinterpreted our model in the same way as so many others have. The implication I perceive is that we believe people are not involved in what they are doing, i.e. they are faking or dissimulating. Such an interpretation is unfortunate from our point of view because it is not at all our intention. What seems to happen is that role metaphor is easily reified by many persons. The proposition of role theory – 'it's as if people may be viewed as actors in a drama' is reduced to, 'people are acting not really living.' In social psychology investigators do not seem to lose the 'as if' characterization of the drama metaphor, but in the area of hypnosis, probably because hypnosis has been associated with sham behaviour, con-artists and quacks as you point out, legitimate investigators seem defensive and over-respond to anything which could suggest that fakery is involved.[7]

Another influential 'non-state' theorist who takes an extreme position in challenging the conventional view that hypnosis can best be understood as an altered state of awareness is T. X. Barber. He is so sceptical about the usefulness of the term that he commonly writes 'hypnosis' in quotation marks, and he deals with the problem of accounting for the inhibition of pain by hypnotic suggestion in various ingenious ways. First, he maintains that surgery is not so painful as is commonly supposed, and that maximum pain is experienced when the skin is cut.[8] It is indeed true that many internal organs are not especially sensitive to cutting, although they are painful when stretched, but as surgical operations normally involve cutting through the skin, this argument is not particularly relevant. Barber argues that we simply do not know whether the operations performed under hypnosis or mesmerism would have been painful if they had been performed without attempting to hypnotize or mesmerize the patient. He quotes some early instances in which surgery was carried out without any hypnotic, mesmeric or chemically induced analgesia, yet the patient appeared to suffer no great pain. Such an instance is that reported by Freemont-Smith in which a woman in the earlier part of the nineteenth century had a breast removed without any analgesic aid. She surprised the gathering in the operating theatre by tolerating the operation with calmness, and after having been bandaged up, thanked the surgeon with a curtsey and walked from the room.[9] This episode certainly demonstrates that some patients can tolerate surgery without much overt pain, but the bulk of evidence indicates that in the period referred to patients suffered a very great deal when operated upon. Such rare instances cannot be used very tellingly to make a general point, and indeed Barber's general line of argument would imply that, for all we know, the chemical anaesthetics which are commonly used today may be quite unnecessary, for the patients *might* not suffer any pain if the surgeon proceeded without them!

It is easy to hold up Barber's case to ridicule for he grasps at every shred of evidence which throws doubt on the effectiveness of hypnotic suggestion as an agency for producing hypnotic analgesia. He mentions, for instance, the nineteenth-century doctor Bernheim and states that, 'The data are generally in line with Bernheim's observation that "hypnotism only rarely succeeded as an anaesthetic"'.[10] But here Bernheim was not referring to his own clinical observations: the (mis)quotation is lifted from the following passage:

Surgeons, especially, sought for an anaesthetic agent in hypnotism, capable of replacing chloroform, and a satisfactory observation (on the incision of the ischio-rectal abscess by Broca and Follin) was presented to the Academy of Science in 1859. Some years afterward,

Dr Guérineau, of Poitiers, announced to the Academy of Medicine that he had amputated the thigh under hypnotic anaesthesia (*Gazette des hôpitaux*, 1859). . . . [Then follow five more accounts of major surgery performed painlessly with hypnotic suggestion.]

In spite of these fortunate trials, surgeons soon showed that hypnotism only rarely succeeds as an anaesthetic, that absolute insensibility is the exception among hypnotizable subjects, and that the hypnotizing itself generally fails in persons disturbed by the expectation of an operation.[11]

Bernheim's main point was that hypnotically-induced analgesia was inferior to that produced by chloroform, *because all subjects are not equally susceptible to hypnosis*. He explains this point earlier in the same book:

More or less complete suggestive anaesthesia or analgesia may be met with in all degrees of hypnotism. It is generally more frequent and more pronounced in instances of the degrees last mentioned: those in which there is deep somnambulism and where there is great aptitude for hallucinations. . . .

In a certain number of cases then, the hypnotic insensibility is complete enough to enable the most difficult surgical operations to be performed. But this is not true of the majority of cases. Hypnotism cannot be generally used as an anaesthetic in surgery; it cannot take the place of chloroform.[12]

The fact is, then, that hypnotic suggestion is unsuitable not because it is unreliable, sometimes succeeding and sometimes failing, but because it is not suitable for *all* people as chloroform and other chemical anaesthetics are.

In spite of Barber's debating techniques and his tendency to over-state his case, his hypercritical attitude is on the whole salutary in enabling us to arrive at a balanced view of what can be done in the alleviation or abolition of pain by hypnotic techniques, and of how the hypnotic mechanisms work. Too many writers have tended to portray hypnosis as though it were a sort of magic which has the power to abolish pain, and given the impression that no sort of scientific inquiry was either necessary or possible.

Differences Between Mesmerism and Hypnotism

Before discussing in detail theories of the mechanisms by which pain can be inhibited by hypnosis, it is necessary clearly to distinguish between hypnosis and mesmerism. Some authors appreciate this, at least with respect to the inhibition of pain. Thus Shor writes:

> A consideration of the historic development of the issue makes it clear that Esdaile and the other mesmerists in the mid nineteenth-century did not induce hypnotic anaesthesia in the modern sense. . . . Using mesmeric passes and relying on preformed expectations of influence rather than verbal suggestion, they very slowly induced a state of profound stuporous slumber.[13]

However, many other authors simply assume that mesmerism (or 'animal magnetism') and hypnosis are identical, an assumption which leads to some confusion. This confusion was natural in the late nineteenth century when hypnotism had not been subjected to much investigation by scientific methods, but many modern writers simply copy the older pundits, particularly with regard to the production of analgesia. Thus Hilgard writes, 'In those days hypnosis was called animal magnetism. . . .'[14] Barber *et al.* also make this false identification, stating, 'If we look at the early reports of painless surgery under mesmerism or hypnotism, we find that, although the procedures apparently reduced anxiety and fear, the extent to which they reduced pain as a sensation may have been exaggerated.'[15] Chertok *et al.* also write as though the difference between mesmerism and hypnotism was simply a change of name: 'On April 12, 1829, Jules Cloquet operated on a cancer of the breast under "magnetic" anaesthesia (the term hypnosis was not introduced until 1843).'[16] But Cloquet was using traditional mesmerism and not hypnotism.

Let us look first at what mesmerists do and then compare their techniques with those of hypnotists. Mesmer himself resorted to many different practices, with the apparent object of provoking a hysterical crisis in his patients. As Sarbin and Anderson remark, 'The "crisis" behaviour observed by Mesmer is *not* the behaviour we now regard as hypnotic.'[17] The practice that later came to be called mesmerism has been described by many authors, and it does not accord entirely with Mesmer's own practices, which involved a wand, a *baquet* and music. Reviewing the mesmeric practice of Esdaile in India, the contemporary Government observers wrote in their Report:

> The patient lay on his back, the body naked from the waist upwards, and the thighs and legs bare; the mesmerizer seated behind him at the head of the bed, leaning over him, the faces of both nearly in contact, the right hand being generally placed on the pit of the stomach and passes made with one or both hands along the face, chiefly over the eyes. The mesmerizer breathed frequently and

gently over the patient's eyes, lips and nostrils. Profound silence was observed. The processes were continued for about two hours each day in ten cases, for eight hours in one case in one day, and for six hours in another case, without interruption. Three cases in the ten were dismissed without satisfactory effect.[18]

In his manual *Practical Instructions in Animal Magnetism* Deleuze describes the long, rhythmic passes that were made over the prostrate body of the subject, passes that were supposed to 'magnetize' him just as a bar of iron is magnetized by stroking it in one direction with a magnet.[19] Topham, a barrister who also practised mesmerism, describes in detail how he mesmerized James Wombell on successive days over a period, so that eventually the surgeon, W. Squire Ward, was able to amputate his leg without pain, the patient lying in a peaceful trance.[20] Esdaile insists that his practice of mesmerism, described above, was carried out *without* explaining to the patients what was to be done to them, and hence the dramatic change in their physical state and mental awareness was due to the physical manipulations performed rather than to any psychological phenomena of expectancy. We may doubt, in fact, whether Esdaile was correct in claiming that none of his patients knew what to expect, for the traditional practices of *Jar Phoonk* (literally stroking and blowing) were well-known in India, and it is probable that Esdaile learnt his mesmerism from his Indian orderlies, rather than from the English mesmerists as he claimed.[21]

The various surviving accounts of nineteenth-century mesmeric practice make several things clear. The patient was immobilized in a recumbent position for rather a long time, and subjected to continuous, rhythmic stimulation from the passes of the mesmerist's hands. The stroking movements were applied to head, trunk and arms, and sometimes went down the legs, as in the 'long pass'. This monotonous process was kept up in silence until the patient eventually showed certain signs, such as non-reaction to pinches and pricks, that the experienced practitioner could detect. According to Elliotson,[22] although the mesmeric trance would remain undisturbed by procedures which would normally be exceedingly painful, it might be broken if one attempted to engage the mesmerized subject in conversation. Evidence on this last point is very contradictory, as will be discussed. The mesmeric trance was self-limiting, the subject arousing himself after a period of quiescence; alternatively the trance might develop into a natural sleep.

The foregoing facts about the induction and nature of the mesmeric state make it quite clear that it is radically different from hypnosis as it has been practised for the past century. Hypnosis is induced by talking to a person and encouraging his imagination to work on suggested ideas. The subject reacts best if he is fully informed about what will happen, and if he actively co-operates in accepting the suggestions that are proposed to him. He tries to imagine and feel what the hypnotist suggests. Typically, the hypnotist uses the metaphor of sleep in inducing the trance, but not invariably; some hypnotists such as Vingoe advocate the induction of what they call an 'alert trance'.[23]

Unlike the induction of the mesmeric state, hypnotism is relatively rapid, and is accomplished in minutes rather than in hours. The hypnotized subject can be engaged in conversation, and he will perform meaningful tasks without disturbance of the trance, in contrast to the stupor which characterizes the mesmeric state. There is no reason, of course, why mesmerism and hypnotism should not co-exist, and undoubtedly in striving to 'magnetize' their subjects, the mesmerists would effectively hypnotize individuals of a specially susceptible nature. One of the early records of a subject showing all the classic signs of hypnotic somnambulism is that of De Puységur's transactions with his servant Victor Race.[24] Victor Race's behaviour when in this state had little resemblance to that of a person in a stuporous mesmeric trance.

Perhaps the most significant difference between mesmerism and hypnotism is in the fact that the former produces a natural general analgesia, but hypnotism *per se* confers no immunity from pain, unless it is specifically and insistently suggested, and a negative hallucination (or, in other words, a hallucination for its absence) for it is carefully worked up. This difference needs some elaboration, for many people believe, against all the experimental evidence, that hypnosis confers an automatic analgesia. In fact, the analgesia which can be produced in hypnosis occurs only where the hypnotist specifies that it will occur, and takes appropriate measures to manipulate the subject's imagery to this end. Typically, the analgesia is local and circumscribed; thus if hypnotic suggestion renders the right hand numb, the rest of the right arm, and of course the left hand, are quite unaffected. Hypnotically-induced analgesia has something in common with those peculiar states of loss of feeling in a part sometimes met with in conditions of conversion hysteria, for instance 'glove anaesthesia'.[25]

In terms of the pain that can be produced experimentally in the laboratory for purposes of research, it has been demonstrated that deeply hypnotized subjects are just as sensitive to it as when they are in the waking state. This was shown by Hilgard with eight very good hypnotic subjects who volunteered to endure a strong pain in the right arm, achieved by immersing it in circulating freezing water. When the negative hallucination was induced in hypnosis, however, they reported that they experienced no pain.[26]

It is important to remember here that pain inflicted in an experimental laboratory on a willing volunteer is different in a number of ways from pain experienced in accidents and in the course of surgery. In the laboratory, there is very much less anxiety, for the experimental subject knows that he will come to no harm; he will not be mutilated or forced to bear more pain than he is willing to accept. In the case of an accident or in surgery this is not so, and a large component of anxiety and general psychological distress is part of the experience, greatly contributing to the intensity of suffering. It has been shown, in fact, that whereas placebos can reduce post-operative pain by as much as 35 per cent, placebo action has very little effect on the experience of pain administered in the experimental laboratory. According to Beecher, placebos relieved only 3 per cent of 173 subjects in experimental studies.[27] The action of a placebo is entirely psychological and it serves to relieve the anxiety component of pain. Hypnosis, therefore, even without specific suggestions for analgesia, can act as a placebo and reduce anxiety in clinical cases, thereby relieving pain to some degree. It has sometimes been used in casualty departments in this manner,[28] and it may be used pre-anaesthetically to calm anxious patients as an alternative to administering drugs.[29] Bartlett[30] has described studies comparing the effect of administering various drugs with the use of hypnosis on surgical patients and has noted the superior performance of the hypnotized patients both pre- and post-operatively with regard to a reduced need for narcotics and a more rapid recovery. The earlier remarks about hypnosis having no intrinsic power to inhibit the mechanisms of pain, must therefore be modified by the admission that, in appropriate circumstances, it may have the power to relieve anxiety and therefore reduce pain. With mesmerism, however, there is reason to believe that it may have a more direct influence on pain mechanisms, even in the presence of high anxiety.

It seems reasonable to regard the mesmeric state as one which is produced by physical manipulations, and characterized primarily by physical phenomena, whereas the hypnotic state is produced by psychological manipulations, and characterized primarily by psychological phenomena. Much of the evidence that we have about mesmerism is confusing because it was not recorded very scientifically, and also, as has been pointed out, mesmerism and hypnotism may occasionally have been co-existent in patients and experimental subjects. Mesmerism may be closely related to a condition studied by animal psychologists known as tonic immobility or 'animal hypnosis'. Most creatures like small mammals and chickens can easily be thrown into this state by putting them in an unaccustomed posture and holding them immobile for a little while. The animal may struggle a little at first, but with gentle though firm restraint will soon become immobile and maintain an apparently stuporous state for some time. Whilst in this state of 'animal hypnosis' it will tolerate pricking or other aversive stimuli without reacting.

The existence of this state was noted long before the time of the mesmerists, one of the early investigators being Daniel Schwenter in 1636. Some modern writers such as Völgyesi[31] and Hoskovec and Svorad[32] have compared the state to human hypnosis, whilst others such as Ratner[33] have been at pains to emphasize the differences between 'animal hypnosis' and human hypnosis. The non-reactivity of animals in this state was well known to the mesmerist Lafontaine, who gave public exhibitions in both France and England, demonstrating how he could throw animals into a trance by making rhythmic mesmeric passes over them and gazing into their eyes. The latter procedure was probably redundant except in so far as it involved restraining and immobilizing the animals for a while. Lafontaine's animals included cats, dogs, lizards, squirrels and, more surprisingly, a lion, and he showed how they would not respond to normally painful stimuli such as pricks in the paws. The analgesic effects of putting animals into a trance have been investigated more recently by Rapson and Jones[34] and by Carli.[35]

The three states of human hypnosis, mesmerism and 'animal hypnosis' are compared in the table below.

	Human Hypnosis	Mesmerism	Animal Hypnosis
Produced by verbal suggestions	Yes	No	No
Provoked by physical stimuli	No	Yes	Yes
Subject non-reactive and stuporous	No	Yes	Yes
Analgesia a natural consequence	No	Yes	Yes
Potentiated by fear	No	?	Yes
Reduced by habituation	No	?	Yes
Evidence for involvement of endorphins	No	?	Yes

While a good deal of research has been done on human hypnosis and 'animal hypnosis' in the present century, there has been virtually no significant body of research into mesmerism, most researchers assuming, as already stated, that it is simply an old name for hypnotism. A few reports relating to mesmerism have appeared in modern times, such as that of Pulos,[36] but in the main we are dependent on various anecdotal accounts from the nineteenth century. The reports of writers such as Elliotson[37] and Esdaile[38] suffer from the fact that they are polemical and written in a climate of acute controversy and ridicule. These authors were also trying to establish a rather preposterous theory of 'magnetism', rather than recording the facts about mesmerism in a detached and scientific manner. Of greater value, though much rarer, are the reports of more objective observers such as those of the official visitors to the Mesmeric Hospital in Calcutta, who gave critical observations of what went on in that hospital, week by week, over a period of six months in 1847.[39]

It will be observed in the table above that we must admit ignorance about mesmerism on three of the seven points. It seems likely, however, that mesmerism is potentiated by fear, for patients awaiting surgical operation in the conditions which obtained in the early nineteenth century would have had good reason to be in a state of acute fear, and this may have made them more susceptible to the influence of mesmerism, if in fact the mesmeric state resembles that which can be produced with animals. Gallup et al.[40] have shown experimentally that the natural response of animals to go into the protective trance is actively potentiated by some additional fear-provoking stimulus, like the presence of a stuffed hawk.

As a condition of fear increases the probability that an animal will show the trance response, it is natural that with repeated attempts to 'hypnotize' them, animals become increasingly less susceptible; they become accustomed to the procedure and less frightened by it. The very reverse happens with human hypnosis: although human subjects do not become very much more susceptible to hypnosis with repeated trials, the tendency is for an increase rather than a decrease in response to be manifested.

Regarding the seventh point in the table, we have no firm evidence about the involvement of endorphins in mesmerism as no research has been done on the question. It is only in recent years that the existence and action of endorphins have been discovered, and still more recently that the secretion of endorphins may be involved in the analgesia shown by 'hypnotized' animals.

As mentioned in Chapter 3, there are substances such as naloxone which act as opioid antagonists, so that when they are injected into the system they cancel the analgesic effect of endorphins. This property has been utilized in experimental work. In a series of experiments with rabbits, Carli[41] showed that the pain-suppressing mechanism present in 'animal hypnosis' could be reduced by the injection of naloxone; thus the implication is that the analgesia is dependent on the presence of endorphins. Similarly, Mayer *et al.*[42] have reported that naloxone reverses the effect of acupuncture analgesia, thus implying that acupuncture needling stimulates the secretion of endorphins. In view of the present confused state of the evidence concerning acupuncture this latter finding should be viewed with some caution. Some recent reports throw a good deal of doubt on the ability of acupuncture to produce any analgesia except through its action as a powerful placebo in people trained to expect such pain reduction.[43]

Experimental Pain and Clinical Pain

Before discussing the possible role of endorphins in the analgesia that can be produced in human subjects by hypnotic suggestion, it is necessary to discuss at some length the general question of laboratory studies of experimental pain. Over the past twenty years Ernest Hilgard and his associates have been investigating the phenomenon of pain produced experimentally in the laboratory and sporadic accounts of such work have appeared elsewhere for a long time. Although a caveat about the relevance of experimental laboratory work to pain encountered in the clinical field has already been made, such work does tell us something about the conditions in which pain can be inhibited by hypnotic suggestion. The conditions in the laboratory may be artificial, but they have the advantage that the exact *quantity* of pain administered can be controlled, and that the same *quality* of pain is experienced by each experimental subject, a feature which is not true of clinical studies.

There are several methods of administering pain in the laboratory,[44] and the results of experiments depend partly on the type of method that has been used. Sharp, sudden pains may be administered by electric shocks; the quantity of the stimulus is carefully graduated and controlled in terms of the voltages used. Of course, a given voltage will not necessarily cause two different people to experience the same amount of pain; each person has to be tested individually to establish what is, for him, a lower threshold (just beginning to be painful) and an upper threshold (an intensity which is utterly unbearable). A personal scale may thus be established for each individual subject.

Other techniques of administering pain include the 'cold pressor test' in which the subject has his forearm immersed in circulating icy water, a procedure which becomes unbearably painful in less than a minute. In this test the objective measure is the length of time the subject is able to tolerate it. A procedure which lasts longer is the induction of ischemic pain: in this, an inflatable cuff is put round the upper arm, as in measuring blood pressure, and when all the blood supply to the lower arm is occluded, a standard amount of muscular effort is performed by the hand. The pain steadily mounts in the arm after the exercise stops, the objective measure again being the time the subject can bear the pain. There are also methods of inflicting experimental pain through mechanical pressure, such as a weight resting on the bony part of a finger. Other experimenters have used the projection of a spot of radiant heat on to the forehead, but this procedure can be dangerous.

Three main indices of the experience of pain can be recorded in the laboratory, the first being physiological signs. It is generally understood that the experience of pain is accompanied by an increase in the pulse rate, increase in electrical skin conductance, rise in blood pressure and increase in the tension of the frontalis muscles of the forehead. All these changes can be monitored by laboratory apparatus.

The second method is by the observation of behavioural signs. Pain is often inferred from behavioural signs such as moaning, flinching, hyperventilation, grimacing and withdrawal from the stimulus. The third method depends upon the subject's own subjective report. He tells you that he is in pain, and he can indicate on some scale the degree to which he is suffering.

All these methods have their deficiencies, and experimenters sometimes confuse the supposed signs of pain with the experience of pain itself. Wyke's warning about confusing epiphenomena with the thing itself in studying pain, has already been quoted in Chapter 3. Indeed, as we have noted, many of the well-known indices of pain apply equally well to its opposite, pleasure. Even such behavioural signs such as flinching are not necessarily indicative of the experience of pain: they may occur if a person anticipates that he may suffer pain.

But with the third indicator of pain, the subjective report, we probably have the most reliable index. Here again it is not infallible; for various personal motives, someone may declare that he is in pain when he is not. Conversely, a person may deny the experience of pain whilst he is really suffering, and it is this possibility that is the chief bugbear of those carrying out research into analgesia. There are, however, techniques for adroitly investigating the honesty of subjects' reports in the laboratory, and these have been discussed by Bowers.[45] Methods have been developed to relate the verbal report of the amount of pain experienced to a physiological index. Thus Hilgard[46] found that both the verbal report of pain on a scale of 0–12, and the measured rise in blood pressure, corresponded very closely during the period that subjects were enduring the cold pressor test.

When a person is hypnotized and given repeated and carefully elaborated suggestions that a part of his body is becoming numb, such a negative hallucination may in fact develop. When questioned, he reports that he has lost all feeling in the part designated. If that part of his body is then subjected to a stimulus that would normally be quite painful, a very curious thing happens. According to the verbal report no pain is being experienced, but according to physiological indices the body is behaving as though it were in pain.[47]

Here we have a conflict of interpretation according to the theoretical stance taken by different investigators. According to role theorists such as Sarbin and Coe, as mentioned earlier, hypnotic analgesia is viewed as in a dramaturgical theoretical model: the discrepancy between report and physiological indices is attributed to the fact that the hypnotized subject is 'really' suffering pain, but in accordance with his total commitment to the role of being in a 'pain-free hypnotic state' he reports that he feels no pain, without any conscious falsehood. Reference has also been made to the highly sceptical theoretical position of Barber, who tends to regard the denial of pain in terms of the sufferer's wish to please the hypnotist. After reviewing some of the literature concerning the experimental studies in which verbal reports and physiological indices of pain were taken with subjects given suggestions for analgesia, Barber commented:

> A substantial number of hypnotic-analgesic and waking analgesic subjects participating in the above experiments manifested physiological responses to pain stimuli which are indicative of anxiety or pain. This raises a crucial question: does the hypnotic analgesic subject undergoing surgery show autonomic responses indicative of anxiety or pain?[48]

There is little information available about the physiological responses of patients undergoing surgery under either hypnotic or chemical anaesthesia. Bowers and Van der Meulen undertook a study concerned with dental surgery, in which patients had hypnotic analgesia alternating with chemical analgesia for identical operations. These authors concluded:

> Across all subjects, the type of analgesia utilized made no difference in the physiological responsiveness of the subjects during this crucial period. In other words, *if* physiological reactivity is viewed as an index of pain, *then* chemical and hypnotic analgesias are equally ineffective in controlling dental pain. Obviously, there is something wrong with this conclusion, since the effectiveness of chemical analgesics is not under question.[49]

We have now discussed laboratory and experimental studies

sufficiently to go back to the question that was raised regarding the final point on our table. Is there evidence bearing upon the question of the involvement of endorphins in hypnotic analgesia? So far, little work has been done on this question as it relates to human hypnosis. Goldstein and Hilgard[50] investigated whether human subjects rendered analgesic by hypnotic suggestion would have this analgesia abolished by the injection of naloxone. The naloxone had no significant effect on their analgesia, thus indicating that the analgesia was not the product of endorphin action. This work needs to be replicated by others, but if it proves to be a reliable finding, it indicates that hypnotic analgesia is caused by a purely psychological mechanism. Thus it is suggested that hypnotic analgesia is wholly a matter of altered processing of information, whereas in 'animal hypnosis', and possibly in mesmerism, physiological blocks prevent the neural impulses reaching the higher centres of the sensorium where they might have been orchestrated into a perception of pain.

The Importance of Individual Differences

In all work with hypnosis, whether it concerns the inhibition of pain, the creation of hallucinations, the generation of amnesia or any of the other classic phenomena, a great deal depends on the subject's susceptibility: enormous differences exist between people as to their degree of response to hypnosis. This fact has been known and studied since the time of Bernheim. That it is not always recognized is due partly to the existence in the clinical field of many practitioners who make their living through hypnotherapy. They are loath to admit that a certain proportion of fee-paying patients are not suitable for the type of therapy which they offer. Furthermore some professional hypnotists, out of personal vanity, like to claim that they can hypnotize anyone, a claim that is by no means justified by the findings of research.

Another reason underlying the attempt to minimize the importance of individual differences in susceptibility to hypnosis concerns the theoretical stance of some modern 'non-state' theorists who place all the emphasis on *what is done* to the subject, rather than making due allowance for his own individual personality characteristics which determine the extent of his ability for hypnotic experience. This difference of emphasis among theoreticians was discussed at the beginning of this chapter.

In general, it is found that the more susceptible people are to hypnosis, the more effective will be the suggestions for analgesia when they are hypnotized. As we have seen, with highly susceptible subjects the analgesia may be so complete that surgical operations can be performed on them without pain. In experimental work, and very occasionally in clinical studies, fairly precise measurements of individual susceptibility are taken using one of a number of standard scales. Perhaps the best known is the Stanford Hypnotic Susceptibility Scale, on which subjects are scored on a twelve-point scale.[51] Such susceptibility scores are quite reliable over time, in that anyone will achieve very much the same score when tested on different occasions, just as he will score much the same IQ on re-testing.

Hilgard and Morgan have published figures relating to pain reduction on the cold pressor test showing that the amount of analgesia obtained was highly related to the subjects' degree of measured hypnotic susceptibility. The figures, relating to results obtained from a group of fifty-four college students of limited hypnotic experience, are shown below.[52]

Level of hypnotic susceptibility		Percentage of pain reduction		
		0 – 10	10 – 32	33+
High	(No. = 15)	7	26	67
Medium	(No. = 23)	26	57	17
Low	(No. = 16)	56	31	13

Similar figures might be shown for studies in the clinical field where hypnotic analgesia has been used effectively for patients suffering from cancer, and in connection with obstetrics, surgery and dentistry.[53] Regrettably, clinicians seldom go to the trouble to measure the differential susceptibility to hypnosis among their patients on standard scales of measurement, even when they are carrying out planned prospective studies. Frequently they rely on their fallible clinical judgement and assign patients to categories of high, medium and low impressionistically. It is this continued disregard for the more rigorous aspects of scientific measurement among medical men and dentists who practise hypnosis that is partly responsible for the continued neglect of hypnosis by researchers into problems of pain.

Some people who are very critical of the studies involving the inhibition of pain by hypnosis, make much of the fact that even among people who are rated rather low on hypnotic susceptibility, a few can achieve some degree of analgesia when it is suggested to them, and that among those who are rated quite high on hypnotic susceptibility, there are a few who fail to achieve much analgesia upon suggestion.[54] But these facts merely emphasize that the relationship between measured susceptibility and a successful response to suggested analgesia, is complex and by no means perfect. Nevertheless, the data from quite a number of studies, both experimental and clinical, confirm that the relationship is as one would expect.

It is still something of a mystery why people vary so greatly in their degrees of hypnotizability. It is a personal characteristic which seems to be a most enduring trait. Although many researchers have directed their attention to this problem and advanced a number of interesting hypotheses about it, there is still no generally accepted explanation for the differences between individuals in this respect. People have undertaken courses of training to increase hypnotic susceptibility, but the amount by which it can be increased is not great.[55]

The Hidden Observer

Experimental work on the inhibition of pain by hypnotic suggestion has produced some surprising results. Some rare individuals are able to exhibit a curious phenomenon known as dissociation. Under special circumstances, including hypnosis, they can carry out activities of which they are not wholly aware, at least in terms of their manifest consciousness. Such dissociation of consciousness is displayed in automatic talking and automatic writing. The dissociated person may say things which are out of keeping with what he is doing and then show no memory for what he has said. Similarly, he may write passages, and then show no memory for what he has written, and deny authorship of it. Such activity may appear to the sceptical as the grossest form of play-acting, but there does appear to be good reason for supposing that it is a genuine phenomenon, and that the hypnotized person who displays such dissociation is operating with his consciousness divided into more than one exclusive sub-system.[56]

Efforts have been made to get dissociated hypnotic subjects to report on their experience at more than one level of consciousness. Kaplan[57] experimented with a subject who was capable of automatic writing under hypnosis. When the subject had achieved a state in which he accepted suggestions for analgesia, and claimed that he felt no pain, Kaplan got the subject's 'hidden observer' to report on his 'true' experience by means of automatic writing. The subject accompanied his verbal report that there was no pain with the written words: 'Ouch, damn it, you're hurting me!' Too much should not be made of this and similar anecdotes, but such findings have been common enough to lead to their being investigated systematically.

The general method employed has been to test the hypnotized subject for analgesia after suggestions, by applying a noxious stimulus and asking for his report, then to tell him that what he is aware of is only part of the information that he is processing. He is told that part of him is more aware of his total experience than is conveyed in his report. This is plausible to the hypnotized subject because he is dimly aware that things are going on outside the focus of his attention; for example, he is aware only of what the hypnotist is saying, even though other people in the room may also be talking.[58]

To gain access to the 'hidden consciousness' (if it exists), the hypnotist says that he will place his hand on the subject's shoulder, as a sign that a 'secret' conversation may take place with the so-called 'hidden observer'. He says that when he removes his hand from the subject's shoulder, everything will be as it was and that the subject will not remember what conversation took place until memory is restored after the hypnosis is ended.

This procedure may seem somewhat preposterous to the sceptic, who will find it difficult to believe that within hypnosis there may be independent and isolated layers of consciousness, between which a subject can be induced to alternate at will. Nevertheless, there are reasonable grounds for supposing that it may be a genuine phenomenon. Some evidence comes from the study of simulators of hypnosis. Such simulators are experimental subjects who have been found, on testing, to be particularly insusceptible to hypnosis, and are then asked by one experimenter to simulate hypnosis with another experimenter who is unaware of the fact. The second experimenter is allocated, in random order, some subjects who are genuinely susceptible to hypnosis and some who are deliberately simulating, and he tries to discriminate between the two groups.[59] It has been found that subjects simulating hypnosis do not give a typical performance when the 'hidden observer' technique is used.[60]

Assuming then, that the 'hidden observer' is a genuine phenomenon representing a level of consciousness different from both waking consciousness and from the level of consciousness of the hypnotized subject, what does he report about his experience of pain when a severe noxious stimulus is applied and he has been rendered apparently analgesic to it by suggestion? The results of a long series of experiments reported by Hilgard and his associates indicate that the 'hidden observer' does indeed report an experience of pain which the hypnotized consciousness denies. The *intensity* of the pain reported, as expressed on a graduated scale, is somewhat less than that reported in a normal waking state.[61]

Before discussing the implications of these experiments, we will turn to some interesting work in the clinical field reported by Chertok *et al*.[62] These authors report on the cases of two women, both of whom had surgical operations with hypnotically suggested analgesia and no medication. The first patient, Mrs D., who had surgery on both a hand and a wrist, was re-hypnotized over two months after the operation and given three successive suggestions under hypnosis, each one requiring an answer. These suggestions are quoted verbatim:

(1) You are back in the operating theater. You are conscious of what is going on around you. You will tell me about it.

(2) You are becoming conscious of your bodily sensations during the operation. You will describe them to me, and tell me what you are thinking at the time.

(3) Even if it seems to you right now that you are not conscious of these bodily sensations, one part of yourself is in fact aware of them. You will gain access to that consciousness, and you will be able to describe these sensations.[63]

On being given suggestion (1) she recalled the presence of many people, being placed on the operating table and talking to the psychologists and medical staff present. All her recollections corresponded with fact. On suggestion (2) she said:

In my arms I felt nothing. I didn't feel a thing for several days. One is quite numb. It doesn't seem any more that it's your own hand they are operating upon. I didn't look, but if I had I'd have felt they were operating on someone else, but not me.[64]

When they proceeded to suggestion (3), which corresponds to eliciting a report from the 'hidden observer', Mrs D. said:

One's whole body is numb, but at the place of the operation it burns at first – like a cut with a penknife. It doesn't last long. Later it burns, it burns! Maybe it's the thermocautery – I didn't see . . . or when they removed the cyst. It burns terribly – as much as the incision. . . . One can bear it. Then it's like hot flushes – it gets worse and worse, and then passes off; it doesn't last. And then you don't feel anything more. So I can't really compare it . . . I didn't see.[65]

The second patient, Mrs T., was subjected to severe dental surgery under hypnotically-suggested analgesia with no medication. Half an hour after the operation she was re-hypnotized, and in reply to suggestion (2) she denied having experienced any sensations of pain, but mentioned the whirring of the dental drill. When given suggestion (3) she said:

As I was relaxed, I wasn't at all afraid of the operation. I cannot say I felt pain. I'm trying to remember, but – yes there were . . . two or

three slight sensations . . . not really painful . . . more like a slight
tickling of the jaw, but I can't even call it pain.[66]

Three days after the operation Mrs T. was interrogated for a second
time under hypnosis. On suggestion (1) she talked about what had
happened before the operation, pointing out that she had had no
anticipatory anxiety. On suggestion (2) she again mentioned the sound
of the drill, and said that she had some sensation of heat. When asked
whether she felt a burn, she denied actually feeling burnt but said that
she had the sensation of heat on her face and said that she was not sure
whether it was in her mouth. She also mentioned little twinges in the
jaw, but again denied that the procedure was painful. On suggestion
(3) she repeated much of what she had said before, but made a remark
about the lady dentist who was treating her that is of great significance
for understanding the nature of hypnotic analgesia. She said:

So she started to treat my tooth, but it was as if she was doing it to
someone else, not to me. I asked myself, 'which tooth is it that she's
treating?' – and I thought, 'all the same, I would like to know which
tooth it is, so that I can keep track and get some idea whether it hurts
or not'. . . . But I didn't feel a thing. . . . I'm trying to understand
why I feel that this work is being carried out on someone else. It's as
if it were another person, but inside me all the same, on whom she's
operating. So that I'm almost like a spectator.[67]

When asked about what this 'second person' felt, the patient replied,
'Of course she was saying: "It hurts! You're hurting me!"' Thereupon
it was suggested that she would no longer be Mrs T., but this second
person who was in pain. The patient (speaking in the person of what
Hilgard would call the 'hidden observer') replied:

Oh it hurts a bit but it's nothing terrible. At times you touched with
your instrument a sensitive place which hurt me, but it didn't
last. . . . Oh, I was probably exaggerating when I said you had hurt
me. It was sensitive but not painful. . . . You were treating a tooth
on the right side, but it's not at all the same as when you gave me
dental treatment in your surgery . . . one can't even compare the
pain . . . it's really like a rather remote pain, which doesn't reach
anything . . . it doesn't seem actually to reach the body, one's own
body. . . . I think that all in all things went very well.[68]

Here we have the same conflict of testimony; the hypnotized Mrs T.
stated that the operation did not hurt at all, but when pressed as to
what 'a second person' might be feeling, she used the significant words,

'Of course, *she* was saying it hurts.' This suggests that she was *attributing* an expression of feeling to this postulated 'hidden observer', and when further pressed she elaborated on it. Since the patient is invited to comment on what this 'observer' must be feeling, it is not unnatural that (knowing what was being done to 'her') the experience of a feeling of pain would be attributed to this postulated second person. A deeper understanding of this curious situation is to be found in a field of psychology known as *attribution theory*[69] which is too elaborate to be discussed here. Kenneth Bowers[70] has discussed the relevance of attribution theory to the experience of hypnotized subjects most insightfully.

Referring back to the experiments of Hilgard and his colleagues, it is natural to assume that when the 'hidden observer' is induced to speak (or write) he is giving an account of what is 'really' being experienced. But this is an unwarranted assumption, for there is no reason to suppose that the report of pain is any 'truer' than the report of analgesia. It is possible that the hypnotized person, having been confidently assured that such a secondary consciousness exists, strives to conform, and so gives an alternative version of what he thinks he must be experiencing. The most obvious alternative report would be to comment on the physiological events in his body, the quickened heartbeat, the altered breathing, the sweating skin, and in the circumstances to label them 'pain', although he is not really having a painful experience. In another context, he might label it as 'pleasure', e.g. when he was experiencing these identical physiological signs, simultaneously with caresses from an attractive partner. We need not necessarily agree with Hilgard's concept of a dissociated personality, but instead explain the secondary report as being the logical result of the hypnotized subject's attempt to conform with a rather odd demand made by the hypnotist. Such an alternative view would also fit the events reported in the clinical case studies of Chertok *et al.*

Yet another explanation of the 'hidden observer' phenomenon might be advanced. When the critical signal takes place – the placing of a hand on the hypnotized subject's shoulder to activate the 'hidden observer' – the subject is aroused to some degree from his hypnotic trance and hence experiences and reports on an experience of pain. When the hand is removed he sinks back gratefully into deep trance, and the suggestion of analgesia is reasserted. This view of the phenomenon would explain why the report of pain refers to an intensity intermediate between the waking experience and that of hypnotic analgesia.

A great deal of space has been devoted to discussing the 'hidden observer' phenomenon because it is crucial to understanding that hypnotic analgesia is not mere play-acting. Two explanations have been offered alternative to that of Hilgard's model of the dissociated consciousness, and neither of them suggests that we should view the phenomenon with disbelief.

Distractors and Information Processing

It has been proposed in this book that the mechanism of hypnotic suggestion is to alter the information-processing system so that incoming stimuli are orchestrated partly in accordance with the stimuli initiated by the hypnotist. This means that the pattern of stimuli which would normally be orchestrated into a percept of pain does not take on that *gestalt*[71] owing to the intruding hypnotist-originated stimuli. The analogy of music has been suggested in this connection; a certain pattern of sounds may be perceived as a harmony until extra sounds are added and the altered pattern is then perceived as a discord.

If this is the mechanism whereby hypnotic suggestion overcomes pain, it should follow that events other than hypnosis may also fulfil the conditions for overcoming pain by psychological means, and this is indeed found to be the case. In the chapter discussing the nature of pain it was pointed out that concurrent experiences such as violent athletic endeavour, or the excitement of the battlefield, or ecstasy of making love can sometimes provide the extra input of stimuli that will negate the perception of pain. Such extra stimuli may be regarded as 'distractors'.

Even quite mild distractors will inhibit pain, provided it is not too intense. Barber,[72] experimenting with student nurses, had them listen to a taped reading of what purported to be the erotic adventures of a certain film star; during the reading a mildly painful stimulus was applied to them. Their report of pain was significantly lower than that of a control group of nurses who had not had the benefit of the distracting tape. The analgesic effect of the distractor worked equally well whether or not the nurses had previously listened to a hypnotic induction patter; indeed, there seems no reason to suppose that the erotic effect of the tape would be enhanced if some of the nurses had been in any way hypnotized previously, for the erotic implications of the tape were not given as hypnotic suggestions. This experimental study tells us something of the power of distractors, but the fact that one sub-group of nurses had previously listened to an induction patter, rather confuses the issue with respect to the power of hypnotic suggestion to attenuate pain.

Perhaps the most interesting example of the inhibition of pain by distraction is the case of acupuncture. It is not argued here that acupuncture acts *solely* as a distractor, indeed, earlier in this chapter reference was made to the possibility that acupuncture needling might cause the secretion of endorphins. But acupuncture must necessarily act as a distractor because the needles are generally inserted at various places *distant* from the part of the body where the pain is, and then twirled manually or vibrated electrically. The needles cause a certain amount of local pain, and, as described by McGarey, 'a deep but minimal aching sensation is often felt when the needles are properly placed'.[73] These aching sensations are not an acute pain, but for analgesia it is necessary for them to build up, and the treatment is started some twenty minutes before surgery is to take place. As well as the deep ache, the needles' vibration produces muscular twitches and contractions which add a proprioceptive component to the pattern of the resultant stimulation.

When discussing the physiology of the production of pain, we considered gate control theory and the possibility that stimulation of large-diameter nerve fibres would inhibit the neural impulses from small-diameter fibres which conduct messages concerned with pain, such inhibition taking place at the postulated spinal 'gate'. Melzack has suggested that acupuncture may indeed fulfil this function, and may be regarded as a special case of hyperstimulation analgesia. According to Melzack:

The stimulation of particular nerves or tissues by needles could bring about an increased central biasing mechanism, which would close the gates to inputs from selected body areas. The cells of the midbrain reticular formation are known to have large receptive fields . . . and the electrical stimulation of points within the central tegmental tract-central grey area can produce analgesia in a half or quadrant of the body. . . . It is possible, then, that particular body areas may project especially strongly to some reticular areas, and these, in turn, could bring about a complete analgesic block in a large part of the body.[74]

We should note, in passing, that the general model of gate control theory referring to efferent stimuli creating a spinal block locally, does not apply generally to acupuncture, for the needling may be done on the face or ears where spinal nerves are not involved. One can, of course, postulate other 'gates', say in the thalamus. However, in the passage quoted above Melzack has referred the postulated 'central biasing mechanism' as being the key factor in acupuncture analgesia. He states elsewhere; 'It is most likely, therefore, that both spinal and supraspinal mechanisms mediate the complex effects of intense stimulation on pain.'[75]

It is not proposed to criticize Melzack's theory of pain inhibition by means of acupuncture; he agrees that acupuncture acts as a distractor, and merely offers a fairly elaborate explanation of how it works. We have been concerned to discuss various examples of the inhibition of pain by distraction, in order to clarify the point of view that hypnosis is not merely a distractor when it is used to inhibit pain. The essential quality of hypnotic suggestion is its meaningful verbal content; because human beings are so powerfully influenced by words it is suggested that it does not matter whether or not the neural stimuli coming from damaged areas are blocked at spinal or thalamic 'gates'. What is controlled is the processing of these stimuli so they do not build up into a percept of pain. The block is psychological rather than physiological.

Again we must go to the analogy of hysterical disorder, and mention that in hysterical blindness or hysterical deafness it is nowhere suggested that there is any block in the optic nerve or auditory nerve: the failure of perception is attributed wholly to a lack of the usual processing of the stimuli projected to cortical sites.

Summary and Conclusion

In summary, it may be stated that the practices of verbal suggestion which have been used for the past century under the general name of hypnotism, when directed to producing an altered state of awareness characterized by various classical phenomena of hypersuggestibility, do not in themselves produce any attenuation of pain. Pain is inhibited only if the hypnotist capitalizes on the subject's high suggestibility and builds up a negative hallucination for pain. In this, hypnotism differs from mesmerism as the latter appears to produce a stuporous state, not unlike that of 'animal hypnosis', in which there is some degree of physiologically produced analgesia. This simple picture is confused by the fact that hypnotism may also act as a placebo, and thus in conditions in which pain is being exacerbated by high anxiety, if the sufferer is prone to react favourably to placebos, the hypnotic state will reduce the experience of pain.

Finally it should be stressed that the power of hypnotism to abolish pain has been greatly exaggerated as well as misunderstood by many professional hypnotists as well as by lay people. People who can calmly endure major surgery with no other analgesic than hypnosis are probably rare in our culture, although most people can benefit to some degree from hypnotic suggestions intelligently directed towards attenuating their experience of pain.

REFERENCES

1 See M. T. Orne, 'Mechanisms of hypnotic pain control', op. cit.; also C. Cedercreutz, R. Lahteenmaki and J. Tulikoura, 'Hypnotic treatment of post-traumatic headache', in J. J. Bonica and D. Albe-Fessard (eds), *Advances in Pain Research and Therapy*, op. cit.

2 H. Bernheim, *Hypnosis and Suggestion in Psychotherapy* (1886), (Trans. C. A. Herter), New York: Jason Aronson, 1973.

3 See E. R. Hilgard, *Hypnotic Susceptibility*, New York: Harcourt Brace & World, 1965.

4 T. R. Sarbin and W. C. Coe, *Hypnosis: A Social Psychological Analysis of Influence Communication*, New York: Holt, Rinehart & Winston, 1972.

5 Ibid., p. 136.

6 E. R. Hilgard, 'Hypnosis and pain', in R. A. Sternbach (ed.), *The Psychology of Pain*, op. cit., p. 236.

7 W. C. Coe, Personal communication dated 13 October, 1978.

8 T. X. Barber, *LSD, Marihuana, Yoga and Hypnosis*, op. cit.

9 F. Freemont-Smith, 'Discussion of Beecher's paper on perception of pain', in *Problems of Consciousness, First Conference*, New York: Josiah Macey Jnr. Foundation, 1950.

10 T. X. Barber, *Hypnosis: A Scientific Approach*, New York: Van Nostrand Reinhold Co., 1969, p. 131.

11 H. Bernheim, op. cit., p. 116.

12 Ibid., pp. 14–22.

13 R. E. Shor, 'Physiological aspects of painful stimulation during hypnotic analgesia', in J. E. Gordon (ed.), *Handbook of Clinical and Experimental Hypnosis*, New York: Macmillan, 1967, p. 554.

14 E. R. Hilgard, 'Hypnosis and pain', op. cit., p. 219.

15 T. X. Barber, N. Spanos and J. F. Chaves, *Hypnosis, Imagination and Human Potentialities*, New York: Pergamon Press, 1974, p. 79.

16 L. Chertok, D. Michaux and M. C. Doin, 'Dynamics of hypnotic analgesia: some new data', *Journal of Nervous and Mental Disease*, 1977, 164, pp. 88–96.

17 T. R. Sarbin and M. L. Anderson, 'Role theoretical analysis of human behaviour', in J. E. Gordon (ed.), *Handbook of Clinical and Experimental Hypnosis*, op. cit.

18 'Report of the Committee appointed by the Government to observe and report on surgical operations by Dr J. Esdaile upon patients under the influence of alleged mesmeric agency', Printed by order of the Deputy Governor of Bengal, Calcutta, 1846. Quoted in *The Zoist*, 1847–8, 5, pp. 51–2.

19 J. P. F. Deleuze, *Practical Instructions in Animal Magnetism*, Part I, (Trans. T. S. Hartshorn), Providence, R.I.: B. Cranston & Co., 1837.

20 W. Topham and W. Squire Ward, 'Account of a case of successful amputation of the thigh during the mesmeric state without knowledge of the patient', Paper read to the Royal Medical and Chirurgical Society of London on Tuesday the 22nd November, 1842, London: H. Baillière, 1842.

21 For an account of Esdaile's probable indebtedness to Indian folk medicine see H. B. Gibson, *Hypnosis: Its Nature and Therapeutic Uses*, London: Peter Owen, 1977, pp. 110–12.

22 J. Elliotson, *Numerous Cases of Surgical Operations Without Pain . . .*, op. cit.

23 F. J. Vingoe, 'The development of a group alert trance state', *International Journal of Clinical and Experimental Hypnosis*, 1968, 16, pp. 120–32.

24 See H. F. Ellenberger, op. cit.

25 See S. B. Guze and M. J. Purley, 'Observations on the natural history of hysteria', *Journal of Psychiatry*, 1963, 119, pp. 260–5.

26 E. R. Hilgard, 'Hypnosis and Pain', op. cit.

27 H. K. Beecher, *Measurement of Subjective Responses*, op. cit.,

28 See L. Goldie, 'Hypnosis in the casualty department', *British Medical Journal*, 1956, 2, pp. 1340–2.

29 See C. T. Mun, 'The use of hypnosis as an adjunct to surgery', *American Journal of Clinical Hypnosis*, 1966, 8, pp. 178–9.

30 E. E. Bartlett, 'Polypharmacy versus hypnosis in surgical patients', *Pacific Medical Journal*, 1966, 74, pp. 109–11.

31 F. A. Völgyesi, *Hypnosis in Man and Animals*, London: Baillière Tindall & Cassell, 1966.

32 J. Hoskovec and D. Svorad, 'The relationship between human and animal hypnosis', *American Journal of Clinical Hypnosis*, 1969, 11, pp. 180–2.

33 S. C. Ratner, 'Comparative aspects of hypnosis', in J. E. Gordon (ed.), *Handbook of Clinical and Experimental Hypnosis*, op. cit.

34 W. S. Rapson and T. C. Jones, 'Restraint of rabbits by hypnosis', *Laboratory Animal Care*, 1964, 14, p. 131–3.

35 G. Carli, 'Animal hypnosis and pain', in F. H. Frankel and H. S. Zamansky (eds), *Hypnosis at Its Bicentennial*, New York: Plenum Press, 1978.

36 L. Pulos, 'Mesmerism revisited', *American Journal of Clinical Hypnosis*, 1980, 22, pp. 206–11.

37 J. Elliotson, *Numerous Cases of Surgical Operations Without Pain . . .*, op. cit.

38 J. Esdaile, *Mesmerism in India and Its Practical Application in Surgery and Medicine*, op. cit.

39 *Report of the Mesmeric Hospital*, op. cit.

40 G. G. Gallup, R. F. Nash, R. J. Potter and N. H. Donegan, 'Effect of varying conditions of fear on immobility reactions in domestic chickens (gallus gallus)', *Journal of Comparative and Physiological Psychology*, 1970, 73, pp. 442–5.

41 G. Carli, 'Animal hypnosis and pain', op. cit.

42 D. J. Mayer, D. D. Price and A. Raffii, 'Antagonism of acupuncture analgesia in man by the narcotic antagonist naloxone', *Brain Research*, 1977, 121, pp. 368–72.

43 See C. Galeano and C. Y. Lueng, 'Has acupuncture an analgesic effect on the rabbit?', *Pain*, 1978, 4, pp. 265–71. See also V. J. Knox and K. Shum, 'Reduction of cold pressor pain with acupuncture analgesia in high and low hypnotic subjects', *Journal of Abnormal Psychology*, 1977, 86, pp. 639–43.

44 See B. Tursky, 'Laboratory approaches to the study of pain', in D. Mostofsky (ed.), *Behaviour Modification and Control of Physiological Activity*, Englewood Cliffs, N.J.: Prentice-Hall, 1976.

45 K. Bowers, *Hypnosis for the Seriously Curious*, Monterey, Calif.: Brooks/Cole Publishing Co., 1976, p. 87.

46 E. R. Hilgard, 'Pain as a puzzle for psychology and physiology', *American Psychologist*, 1969, 24, pp. 103–13.

47 The question of the discrepancy is discussed by J. P. Sutcliffe, ' "Credulous" and

"sceptical" views of hypnotic phenomena. Experiments on esthesia, hallucination and delusion', *Journal of Abnormal and Social Psychology*, 1961, 62, pp. 189-200.

48 T. X. Barber, *LSD, Marihuana, Yoga and Hypnosis*, op. cit., pp. 226-7.

49 K. Bowers and S. J. Van der Meulen, 'A comparison of psychological and chemical techniques in the control of dental pain', Paper delivered to the Society for Clinical and Experimental Hypnosis Convention, Fall 1972.

50 A. Goldstein and E. R. Hilgard, 'Lack of influence of the morphine antagonist naloxone on hypnotic analgesia', *Proceedings of the National Academy of Science* (USA), 1975, 72, pp. 2041-3.

51 A. M. Weitzenhoffer and E. R. Hilgard, *The Stanford Hypnotic Susceptibility Scale: Forms A and B*, Palo Alto, Calif.: Consulting Psychologists Press, 1959.

52 E. R. Hilgard and A. H. Morgan, 'Heart rate and blood pressure in the study of laboratory pain in man under normal conditions and as influenced by hypnosis', *Acta Neurobiologica Experimentalis*, 1975, 35, pp. 941-59.

53 See E. R. Hilgard and J. R. Hilgard, *Hypnosis in the Relief of Pain*, Los Altos, Calif.: W. Kaufmann Inc., 1975.

54 See G. F. Wagstaff, *Hypnosis, Compliance and Belief*, Brighton: Harvester Press, 1981, Chap. 8.

55 See M. J. Diamond, 'Modification of hypnotizability: a review', *Psychological Bulletin*, 1974, 81, pp. 180-98.

56 For early discussions of the concept of divided consciousness see P. Janet, *The Major Symptoms of Hysteria*, New York: Macmillan, 1907; and M. Prince, *The Dissociation of a Personality*, New York: Longmans Green, 1906.

57 E. A. Kaplan, 'Hypnosis and pain', *Archives of General Psychiatry*, 1960, 2, pp. 567-8.

58 See E. R. Hilgard and J. R. Hilgard, *Hypnosis in the Relief of Pain*, op. cit., Chap. 9.

59 See M. T. Orne, 'On the simulating subject as a quasi-control group in hypnotic research: what, why and how?', in E. Fromm and R. E. Shor (eds), *Hypnosis: Research Developments and Perspectives*, Chicago: Aldine-Atherton, 1972.

60 See E. R. Hilgard, J. R. Hilgard, H. MacDonald, A. H. Morgan and L. S. Johnson, 'Covert pain in hypnotic analgesia: its reality as tested by a real-simulator design', *Journal of Abnormal Psychology*, 1978, 87, pp. 655-63.

61 See E. R. Hilgard, H. MacDonald, A. H. Morgan and L. S. Johnson, 'The reality of hypnotic analgesia: a comparison of highly hypnotizables with simulators', *Journal of Abnormal Psychology*, 1978, 87, pp. 239-46.

62 L. Chertok, D. Michaux and M. C. Doin, 'Dynamics of hypnotic analgesia: some new data', op. cit.

63 Ibid., p. 90.

64 Ibid., p. 91.

65 Ibid.

66 Ibid., p. 92.

67 Ibid., pp. 92-3.

68 Ibid., p. 93.

69 See H. Kelley, 'Attribution theory in social psychology', in D. Levine (ed.), *Nebraska Symposium on Motivation*, Lincoln, Neb.: University of Nebraska Press, 1967.

70 K. S. Bowers, 'Hypnosis, attribution and demand characteristics', *International Journal of Clinical and Experimental Hypnosis*, 1973, 21, pp. 226-38.

71 The word *gestalt* implies a recognized configuration of elements appearing in a fixed relationship to one another. It derives from the Gestalt School of psychology.

72 T. X. Barber, 'Effects of hypnotic induction, suggestions of anesthesia and distraction on subjective and physiological responses to pain', cited in T. X. Barber, N. Spanos and J. F. Chaves, *Hypnosis, Imagination and Human Potentialities*, op. cit.

73 W. A. McGarey, 'The philosophy and clinical aspects of acupuncture, from the framework of Western medicine', in *Transcript of the Acupuncture Symposium*, Los Altos, Calif.: Academy of Parapsychology and Medicine, 1972, pp. 12-22.

74 R. Melzack, *The Puzzle of Pain*, op. cit., p. 189.

75 Ibid., p. 184.

6

INDIVIDUAL DIFFERENCES IN
SUSCEPTIBILITY TO PAIN

Early in life we learn how other people react to our outward
expressions of pain. Crying over a grazed knee may bring a welcome
expression of concern and affection from caring adults, and even a
chocolate by way of compensation; but if we cry for too long or too
often, our tears may bring a sharp reproof and an injunction not to be
a silly cry-baby over a little scratch. From time immemorial mothers
have appreciated the laws of operant conditioning governing the
expression and experience of pain which have recently been expounded
so usefully by specialists such as Fordyce.[1] From interaction with our
peers we also learn that there are great individual differences in how
people react to pain-producing experiences. We can never feel
another's pain, but to judge from others' yells, complaints and
flinching, some appear to be more, and some less, susceptible to pain
than ourselves.

Different communities, and indeed, different families, have different
expectations about what is normal in the experience and expression of
pain. In some traditions it is 'girlish' to admit to feeling pain for minor
causes, and boys who cry easily are regarded as 'cissies'. We may be led
to wonder about the mysteries of subjective experience: how much
does our friend experience an event as very painful, and how much is
he just prone to make a fuss?

Cultural Differences

There have been a number of studies of the expression of pain in
different cultural groups. We may assume that, within the individual
differences due to heredity, the child's first reference standard is that of
his family; also there may well be different cultural norms in the
expression of pain. Shoben and Borland[2] found that the attitudes of
different families were highly relevant to how individuals would react
to the threat and the reality of dental pain. Similarly, Johnson and

Baldwin[3] showed that the mothers of children who exhibited excessive fear of dental pain, themselves scored highly for anxiety on a psychological test.

In the USA, that melting-pot of so many cultural groups, family influences are still strong enough to give children different types of upbringing according to their parents' ethnic origins. Yankees, Irish, Jews, Italians, Negroes, Puerto Ricans, Eskimos and American Indians have all been the subject of studies comparing reactions and attitudes to pain. An early study by Zborowski[4] indicated that Yankees have a matter-of-fact attitude to pain, and do not give much outward expression of it publicly. By contrast, according to this study, American Jews and Italians tend to be vociferous in their complaints of pain, and try to elicit the support and sympathy of others.

Three cultural groups, whites, blacks and Puerto Ricans, have been compared in independent studies by Spielberger *et al.*,[5] Corah[6] and Weisenberg *et al.*[7] These studies have all shown the same differences between the groups: Puerto Ricans manifested the most generalized anxiety associated with pain, whites the least, with blacks being intermediate. The Puerto Ricans also showed a pronounced reluctance to face the realities of pain, an attitude shown least by the whites, and intermediately by the blacks.

Studies such as those of Tursky and Sternbach,[8] comparing Yankees, Irish, Italians and Jews, showed significantly different patterns of autonomic response to pain-producing stimuli, which the authors attributed to different cultural attitudes to pain. This, and much other research work on ethnic differences which was conducted up to the 1960s, was later criticized by those concerned to play down all ethnic and cultural differences, for obvious political reasons. Zborowski,[9] in spite of his earlier research, criticized many of the findings as being 'myths', but such studies have still continued. Woodrow *et al.*[10] conducted a huge experimental study with 41,119 individuals, comparing whites, blacks and orientals. Contrary to the old stereotype of the impassive, stoical oriental, they found that whites tolerated pain better, with blacks being intermediate. It should be pointed out that such studies are of relative *tolerance* of pain, and that we cannot generalize from them to assume that these contrasted groups necessarily differed in their *experience* of pain. One wonders too whether the results would have been different if the ethnic group of the experimenters had been systematically varied. Where the studies are clinical (e.g. the 1952 study by Zborowski) we are apt to deduce from the finding that Jews and Italians complain more about pain, that they feel it more, without perhaps taking into account the general attitudes of these cultural groups to matters unconnected with pain. Was the complaining specifically pain-related, for instance, or did those who complained most also create more of a public fuss over such matters as the meals being late or the soup cold?

There have been some studies in which attempts were made to compensate for differences between the cultural or ethnic origins of the experimenter and that of the people studied. For instance, Lambert *et al.*[11] compared eighty Jewish students with eighty non-Jewish students on a pain tolerance test, using both an obviously Jewish and an equally obviously non-Jewish experimenter. The study was further complicated by giving sub-groups of the testees advance information that Jews had been shown to have greater (or lesser) tolerance for pain. As might be expected, these experimental manipulations had some effect on the results of the experiment, but while the study gives information about artefacts of attitude and motivation which are encountered in experimental studies, it can hardly be said to enlighten us much as to whether there are real differences in pain tolerance between Jewish and non-Jewish Americans in everyday life. In terms of hard evidence, the extent to which there are definable individual differences in susceptibility to pain related to cultural and ethnic factors, has yet to be finally determined.

While it is indeed likely that there are significant differences between ethnic groups in the expression of pain because of cultural differences in child-rearing practices and norms of social expression, it is also possible that such differences relate to inherent differences of a neurophysiological nature. We know very little about this, but as will be discussed later, the experience of pain relates to some basic personality parameters which have a biological basis, and there is ample data on the biological differences between the major ethnic groups.

Pain and Personality

In addition to studies of differences between different ethnic and cultural groups in the expression of pain, there has been significant research into the relationship between pain and personality. An early experimental study by Lynn and Eysenck[12] investigated tolerance of pain in relation to the different personality parameters measured by the Maudsley Personality Inventory (MPI). Volunteer subjects were assessed on that psychological test, and subjected to pain produced by a spot of radiant heat projected on to the forehead. The more extraverted subjects were found to be less affected by the aversive stimulus than the introverted; also, the personality trait of neuroticism was significantly related to the results. The more 'neurotic' subjects, as we would expect from our knowledge of the involvement of anxiety in the experience of pain, were less able to tolerate the heat stimulus. The greater pain tolerance of the more extraverted subjects deserves further discussion, and relates to the whole concept of extraversion as a personality trait with an underlying neurophysiological basis.

Diana Haslam[13] compared a group of 'extraverts' with a group of 'introverts' (selected on the basis of their scores on the MPI) and subjected them to the same type of radiant heat stimulus on the forehead that Lynn and Eysenck had used. She was interested not in how much pain they could tolerate, but in the intensity of the heat stimulus which would produce a sensation of pain, that is, in the pain threshold. She found that the extravert group had a higher threshold for pain, a finding that does not have much support from other studies. She then attempted to change the operative extraversion level of the subjects by administering caffeine, a drug that has been shown in various experiments temporarily to introvert the personality (which is why we drink coffee when we wish to concentrate on study). The administration of caffeine citrate in the second part of this study resulted in a significant tendency for the pain threshold to be lowered.

Not all experimental studies have shown clear relationships between the personality traits of extraversion and neuroticism and tolerance for pain. Levine et al.[14] failed to find any such relationship in two separate samples of experimental subjects. Davidson and Bobey, who espouse a sensitizer-repressor explanation of individual differences in suscepti-bility to pain, report, perhaps with some triumph:

> Eysenck (1967) has reviewed some of the supporting literature on the relationship between introversion-extraversion and pain tolerance. Martin and Inglis (1965), in an effort to relate Lynn and Eysenck's (1961) finding to pain tolerance in narcotic addicts found no significant correlation between extraversion and pain tolerance.[15]

Davidson and Bobey do not mention that in the study by Martin and Inglis,[16] one part of the Lynn-Eysenck study was confirmed by a significant negative correlation between pain tolerance and neuroticism; the other part, concerning extraversion, was also confirmed as to tendency, but at a low level of statistical significance. They go on to relate that:

> In an attempt partially to resolve the controversy about the relationship between extraversion and pain tolerance, Davidson and McDougall (1969) obtained pain tolerance measures from female subjects with a heat test and cold pressure [sic] test. Their data showed that neither extraversion nor neuroticism was significantly related to pain tolerance.[17]

This statement is somewhat misleading, for if we look up the publication in question,[18] we find that there was a large and quite extraordinary difference between the extraverts and introverts on tolerance for pain in the cold pressor test, the latter having about seven times greater *variance* of pain tolerance scores! What this remarkable statistic means is anybody's guess.

Laymen may gain some amusement from reading of the theoretical squabbles between scientists who support different theoretical systems, but a bald statement of what people *failed* to find in a particular study is seldom very enlightening; what is of more interest is what they did find, and the details, if they are willing to report them, are often of great interest in revealing what the experimenters have been up to. Popularizers of science such as Eysenck inevitably over-simplify issues to some degree, and hence rouse the ire of those holding to opposing theoretical orientations. Experiments do not always seem to have been designed objectively to clarify a controversy; sometimes they appear to have been designed to prove so-and-so wrong! In the end, it is the bulk of findings arrived at by different people working independently in different research centres which help to settle controversies one way or another, and to develop coherent theories. The remark about Eysenck having reviewed some of the *supporting* literature on the relationship between extraversion and pain tolerance, is in the usual tradition of academic debate; how far it is justified must be determined by reading the book in question.[19]

The negative relationship between extraversion and susceptibility to pain, is generally confirmed in clinical studies. Bond and Pearson[20] divided fifty-two female cancer patients into three groups: group 1 were neither suffering from pain nor receiving analgesic drugs; group 2 were experiencing some pain but had not asked for pain-killing drugs; group 3 experienced pain and demanded pain-killing drugs. Group 1 were somewhat high on extraversion, and remarkably low on neuroticism, as measured by the Eysenck Personality Inventory (a later development of the MPI). Group 2 were low on extraversion and high on neuroticism, and group 3 were high on both extraversion and neuroticism. These somewhat complex results have a perfectly straightforward explanation and illustrate the known relationships between personality and the expression and experience of pain. In all groups higher neuroticism meant more pain; group 3 might appear to be something of an anomaly until we remember that higher extraversion means more demanding behaviour; the neurotic extravert is apt to make relatively more complaints and to demand remedies if he is suffering.

Petrie[21] also found that extraverts experienced less pain than introverts in a clinical study. She studied a population of patients who were recovering from surgery and from bronchoscopy, their degree of pain being assessed by independent ratings made by a physician, a surgeon and a nurse. The patients' degree of extraversion was assessed by the MPI. Comparing patients judged to be suffering least pain with those suffering most (and omitting those in the moderate category), the former group were found to be significantly more extraverted. She did not find any significant difference in the average neuroticism scores of the contrasted groups, which is perhaps surprising. The general findings are that people higher on neuroticism tend to experience more pain, and people higher on extraversion are less susceptible to pain, but if extraverts have to suffer in a clinical situation, they complain more about it.

The Psychiatric Approach

The above findings have been confirmed by studies of psychiatric patients. Thus Merskey[22] found that in a psychiatric population it was the more extraverted patients who complained most about pain. Studies dealing with emotionally disturbed patients diagnosed as neurotic show a high incidence of those reporting pain. Merskey has shown that persistent pain is most frequently associated with neuroses of a more hysterical type, rather than with the more severe conditions of psychosis (insanity). Strangely, conditions of schizophrenia, the illness which temporarily or permanently disorganizes the whole personality, are negatively associated with pain. According to Petrie, 'During this illness a lighted cigarette may be retained in the hand when it is burning the fingers, and severe self-mutilation may be practiced.'[23] Chronic schizophrenics will often tolerate without complaint severe physical diseases which would give rise to pain in normal people.

A good deal of research into the personality characteristics of patients suffering from persistent pain has been carried out with the aid of a psychiatric test known as the Minnesota Multiphasic Personality Inventory (MMPI). This necessitates the patient sorting through a large number of cards, each bearing a statement, and deciding whether the statement is 'true' or 'false' in relation to himself. Analysis of the results of his card-sorting gives a personality profile on a number of descriptive scales which are fairly meaningful with psychiatric patients, but less so when applied to people who are not emotionally disturbed.

The work of Sternbach[24] and others has shown that four types of pain patients may be distinguished according to their personality profiles on the MMPI: 1. Patients who show an extreme preoccupation with physical health, and are high on the *hypochondriasis* scale; 2. those who show a high score on the *depression* scale and admit that their pain condition has 'got them down'; 3. patients who are relatively low on the *depression* scale, but high on both *hypochondriasis* and *hysteria*; 4. those who are high on the *psychopathic deviate* scale. It is suggested by Sternbach that patients in the third group focus on their bodily symptoms in order to avoid suffering from depression, a point of view supported by Pilling et al.,[25] who appear to think that patients choose to experience pain rather than experiencing anxiety and depression. The fourth group are presumed by Sternbach to be using pain symptoms deliberately to manipulate others. This type is said to characterize those who have litigation pending in connection with their injuries.

How useful the MMPI scales are in helping us to understand meaningful differences in pain experience, and in assisting the process of therapy, is a matter of controversy. An intensive study by Jamison *et al.*[26] of fifty-one patients suffering from various forms of chronic pain and attending a pain management clinic, demonstrated that personality profiles on the MMPI were of very little use in predicting the successful outcome of treatment or in aiding the understanding of the patients' troubles. The Eysenck Personality Inventory was also used in this study, but although the results tended to confirm the lower extraversion and higher neuroticism of pain patients, it did not aid in the prediction of success of treatment.

Sternbach,[27] discussing individual differences among his patients, has reported that 'hypochrondriacal' patients do poorly in his treatment programme, but that this may merely mean that they are suffering from painful conditions which have not been properly diagnosed or treated.

The clinical literature shows a number of cases where the patient complained of some persistent pain arising from a condition which doctors were unable to diagnose, and was therefore labelled 'hypochrondriacal'.[28] Yet if any one of us, however well balanced emotionally, were to suffer over a period of time from two or three painful conditions which our medical advisers were incompetent to diagnose, it is likely that we would score highly on the *hypochrondriasis* scale of the MMPI, for we would naturally display 'extreme somatic preoccupation'. Melzack has expressed the position very well:

Treatment may sometimes enhance rather than diminish pain, which may lead to further treatment that may make the patient even worse. We have all seen patients crippled with back pain, who have undergone several disc operations, rhizotomies, cordotomies, and are finally turned over to the psychiatrist. The so-called pain tract was cut, not once but several times, and if the patients are still in pain, they are, by definition in terms of specificity theory, malingerers or neurotics. Small wonder that by this time the patients are depressed, resentful, anxious and attentive to their pain and nothing else.[29]

At the same symposium where Melzack spoke, Taub made a plea against the too easy assumption that chronic pain can be attributed to the patients' psychological state. He said:

The point I want to emphasize is this: is it not possible . . . that these patients, or at least some of them, are suffering from some form of illness, the nature of which we do not know? I think it is most important to use psychophysiological methods for diagnosis and also to realize that there are a great many pain syndromes which are as yet undescribed. The primary function of the pain physician, in addition to treatment, should be the recognition and description of these syndromes.[30]

It is significant that in the study by Pilling *et al.*, cited above, the presenting symptom of the patients was pain; it was the doctors who decided that they were 'psychiatric' cases. It is this tendency of doctors to allocate cases of persistent pain which they cannot properly diagnose to the psychiatric category, that inevitably inflates the percentage of psychiatrically diagnosed patients who complain of pain. (Spear[31] gives a figure of from 40 to 50 per cent.) Nevertheless, it is in keeping with all experience, professional and lay, that emotional disturbance will tend to transform conditions of minor discomfort into persistent pain, and that the painful condition may further exacerbate the emotional disturbance.

Augmenting and Reducing Perception

A highly interesting area of research into individual differences in susceptibility to pain arose originally out of the study of the effects of leucotomy in the 1950s. It has already been mentioned that one of the effects of this neurosurgical operation is that while pain is still experienced in terms of location and intensity, the leucotomized patient no longer experiences the suffering component of the pain in the same way. The operation effectively alters the personality of the patient in an extraverting direction. An early study by Petrie[32] of one hundred leucotomized patients showed that the operation not only reduced their perception of pain, but also altered the measurable personality on a number of traits. The changes were greater after a larger than a smaller incision, and more apparent when it was the dominant rather than the non-dominant half of the brain involved.

The fact that accidental damage or surgery of the frontal lobes of the brain can cause significant changes in personality, has long been recognized. A well-known historical case is that of Phineas Gage, a workman concerned with rock-blasting operations, who had a crowbar driven through the front of his head by an accidental explosion. He survived the accident, but when he had recovered from the wound, his whole personality was seen to have changed. From being steady and conscientious, he became a quite different character, remarkable for his shiftlessness and untrustworthy habits.

For a long time the early researchers who were trying to map out the functions of different parts of the brain, did not know what to make of the frontal lobes, for they did not appear to have any clearly definable function. Work by the neurologist Egas Moniz and the surgeon Almeida Lima on humans in 1936, following previous work that others had done on the brains of animals, suggested that the frontal cortex might be concerned in a rather subtle way with the capacity to plan ahead, and so began the era of tentative surgery with humans whose behaviour was so grossly disturbed that brain surgery seemed justified. One of the main conditions for which leucotomy was used was obsessive compulsive neurosis. In this condition the patient may be so tormented by worry that he commits suicide.

Various types of the operation have been tried, the main feature being the severance of some of the nerve fibres leading up from the thalamus to the frontal lobes. The early promise of the psychosurgery initiated by Freeman and Watts[33] in the 1940s was not fulfilled, and the operation has been rarely performed since the 1950s. Any sort of operation that alters a patient's personality is a drastic last resort, for as well as reducing the patient's propensity to worry too much, various other less desirable consequences may ensue. The personality is changed in a manner similar to alcoholic intoxication; sensitivity to the feelings of others is reduced, crude egotism is increased, together with laziness and lack of any ambition.

Although the operation makes people more indifferent to pain it does not decrease 'sensitivity'; that is, the threshold for the perception of pain is unaltered. The phenomenon which changes is entirely psychological, and is not concerned with sensory acuity.

Petrie describes how her early work in connection with the psychological testing of patients before and after leucotomy operations alerted her to the fact that the study of individual differences in personality had great relevance in the study of pain. She writes:

The implication that certain specific personality characteristics are related to greater tolerance for pain and that these specific characteristics may provide explanatory concepts for such tolerance had begun to concern me earlier. . . . . Numerous additional factors, as well as the observation of many different kinds of patients, led me to seek evidence of the individuality of suffering – of intense and subdued experience in different persons, and in the same person after treatments that increased tolerance for pain – and thus to the concepts of reduction and augmentation.[34]

For her, the concepts of augmentation and reduction are fundamental to the study of individual differences in the experience of pain. The augmentation-reduction continuum refers to a general mode of perception of all stimuli received from the environment. 'Reducers' are people who, at the extreme, hunger for intense stimuli, the volume of which they can easily reduce to manageable and comfortable intensity. To an extreme reducer, the atmosphere provided by a blaring disco is very congenial. Reducers are naturally quite tolerant of pain. 'Augmenters' are people whose basic tendency is to exaggerate the intensity of all the stimuli they receive: thus, at the extreme, they are apt to find their surroundings too bright, noisy, smelly, exciting and painful. Their problem is to protect themselves from the intensity of over-stimulation. People who are intermediate on this continuum are called 'moderates'.

This concept sounds plausible at the level of theory-building, but what factual evidence supports it? The support for it comes from a great body of experimental evidence, some of it antedating Petrie's work, and some later than hers, such as that of Von Knorring[35] and his associates in Sweden using electro-physiological methods of investigation. It can be validated in the study of any perceptual modality.

Research into individual differences in augmentation-reduction has largely used the modality of touch. In the human being there is great sensitivity in the hands as organs of perception of size. If, when blindfolded, we grasp an object between our fingers, we can judge its exact size with a remarkable degree of accuracy. The touch modality lends itself to very accurate measurement of the tendency to under-estimate or over-estimate size under special circumstances, and this tendency can be manipulated by drugs and other experimental procedures. The experimental procedure for testing the individual's augmentation-reduction tendency, as set out by Klein and Krech[36] and adapted by Petrie,[37] is basically as follows.

The subject must first rest his hands for a period of forty-five minutes in order that his sense of touch is not affected by recent tactile experience; he is then blindfolded and asked to feel a rectangular wooden measuring block with his right forefinger and thumb in order to estimate its width. He is then asked to feel with his other hand a long, tapering, wooden block, and to say at which point he feels it to be subjectively equal in width to the measuring block. This measurement is made four times in succession to get an accurate base-line of his subjective estimate.

In the next part of the experiment the subject is given a wider block to feel with his right hand, and he is asked to stroke this for a period of ninety seconds, this tactile stimulation producing an odd 'satiation' of the tactile sense. His subjective estimate of the width of the original measuring block is then tested as before, and thus his tendency to under-estimate, over-estimate or come to the same judgement can be accurately assessed.

There are variations on this basic procedure involving different periods of tactile stimulation and rest, and different sizes of blocks. A photograph of the testing apparatus appears in Petrie's book and is fully explained in her appendix.

The results of such tests show that an extreme augmenter will over-estimate size by as much as 50 per cent after the tactile stimulation, and that an extreme reducer will under-estimate by about the same amount. The individual tendency to reduce or to augment is remarkably constant; that is, if one is a reducer on one occasion it is very unlikely that one will be a moderate or an augmenter on another, when tested under the same conditions. As it is a reliable personal tendency, it is suitable for experimentation in relation to other personality attributes (such as the extent to which an individual is susceptible to pain), and in relation to the degree to which the tendency can be modified by drugs and other variable factors.

Petrie's early work was carried out at the Maudsley Hospital in association with H. J. Eysenck, and was concerned with problems of pain perception and differences in personality. Later she moved to America and worked on this topic with a group of psychologists and medical doctors, relating it to a new and highly interesting area of research: tolerance of *absence* of stimulation or, as named by Bexton et al.,[38] 'sensory deprivation'.

It had been shown that when subjects are isolated in comfortable seclusion, with a very low level of any sort of stimulation, after some hours they begin to experience distress and suffering. Although volunteer subjects may be quite highly paid simply to lie on a couch with masked eyes, hands in soft cuffs and no variable sound, after a time they can stand the absence of stimuli no longer, and they ask to be released from this well-paid isolation. Differences in degree of tolerance for sensory isolation depend upon measurable differences in personality.

Working with Solomon and Collins, Petrie[39] participated in a study in which they recruited nineteen subjects who had already been tested for tolerance of pain, and nine subjects who had been tested for toleration of sensory deprivation. These two groups of subjects were then tested for augmentation-reduction on the tactile apparatus. It was found that those who had the most tolerance for pain showed a significant tendency to *reduce*, and those who had tolerated sensory deprivation longest showed a significant tendency to *augment*. These findings closely paralleled a great deal of experimental work concerning the Eysenckian personality dimension of introversion-extraversion.

Later work concerning the relationship between tolerance for sensory deprivation and tolerance for pain has been ambiguous. Some experimenters (e.g. Zubeck)[40] have found that those who will stay longest under conditions of sensory deprivation will also endure most experimental pain: others (e.g. Minard)[41] have found results which have confirmed Petrie's findings. The outcome of such experimental work is naturally highly affected by situational factors, in that some subjects who are very highly motivated will manage to withstand the utmost pain and also force themselves to endure the distress of staying for a long period in the sensory isolation chamber. As always, we are faced with the ultimate impossibility of measuring the actuality of subjective pain and distress; we can only measure its behavioural results. Zuckerman comes to the reasonable judgement that 'The Petrie hypothesis remains unproven though still promising.'[42]

Drugs and Perceptual Tendencies

That great psychologist P. G. Wodehouse created a character who was alleged to have been born two double whiskies below par. He required these two drinks to bring him up to the level of the normally functioning man. On the basis of general observation, one cannot help but agree with Wodehouse that some individuals do appear to have this disability. Let us see how scientists have set about studying this aspect of human variation, as well as the converse tendency, so well illustrated by other characters in Wodehouse's stories.

The effect of alcohol on the augmentation-reduction tendency has been tested by various researchers. Twenty-seven volunteers, who were not patients, were tested at the Boston Sanatorium by the method described above.[43] Seven of them proved to be augmenters, ten were moderates and ten reducers. Their status on the personality continuum having been established, they were given a drink which either did or did not contain vodka, the tester being kept in ignorance of which drink was being administered, as a precaution against bias.

The overall effect of alcohol on the whole group of volunteers was to increase their tendency to *reduce*. However, when the three sub-groups, augmenters, moderates and reducers, were considered separately, it was seen that the group average was strongly affected by the change in just one sub-group, the augmenters. In this experiment the change following alcohol was quite dramatic, for the augmenters reduced their estimate of size on re-testing proportionately even more than those who were classed as reducers. The alcohol dosage was small, and had very little effect on either the reducers or the moderates.

This study is highly suggestive as to how a drug like alcohol may relieve pain in some people but not in others. If people are suffering from pain because their individual style of perception is to augment the effect of all the stimuli they receive, then alcohol will counteract this augmenting tendency and increase their tolerance of pain. If they are reducers or even moderates, however, the same quantity of alcohol will have little effect on their experience of pain.

The above experiment was repeated with another drug, aspirin, and much the same results were obtained. The reducers and moderates did not change much, but the performance of the augmenters was significantly affected by the aspirin in the direction of reduction. Aspirin is an analgesic drug, but unlike alcohol it is presumed to have little effect on the central nervous system; its effects appear to be on the peripheral nerves. The mechanism by which it would affect perceptual reactivity is not at all clear.

Another drug, chlorpromazine (Largactil), has been investigated with regard to its effect on the augmentation-reduction continuum. This drug is one of the phenothiazines and is classed as one of the major tranquillizers. It is used extensively in the treatment of schizophrenia, where it not only calms the agitated patient but has the additional effect of alleviating the hallucinations and delusions which characterize this condition, putting the patient more in touch with the world around him.

Bradley[44] has characterized chlorpromazine as a drug which makes the individual more sensitive to information coming into the nervous system from the outside, that is, it changes perceptual reactance in the direction of increased augmentation. This would imply that the schizophrenic patient suffers from an extreme perceptual reduction and that chlorpromazine helps him by alleviating this tendency; he does indeed appear to live in a world of his own, isolated from outside stimuli, hence his curious insensitivity to pain.

Seventeen patients at Toronto Psychiatric Hospital who were suffering from schizophrenia were tested on two occasions on the tactile perceptual apparatus.[45] The great majority were found to be reducing, but a minority were found to be unstable, shifting from extreme augmentation to extreme reduction, or vice versa, between the two occasions on which they were tested. This instability of perceptual style is typical of the illness. Although there are many theories of schizophrenia, some of them stressing its biochemical aspects more than others, there is a general consensus that the pre-psychotic personality tends to be that of a rather over-sensitive person, hence the hypothesis that the illness is one of extreme and pathological reaction to over-sensitivity, a withdrawal into extreme perceptual reduction which is maintained rather erratically.

It seems, therefore, that there is an important personality dimension, augmentation-reduction, which can be modified by the administration of drugs. It relates to how each of us experiences the world about us, including the degree to which we experience pain. The work of Petrie, Collins and Solomon showing that greater tolerance of pain was associated with a greater tendency to perceptual reduction, referred to earlier, was confirmed at McGill University by Poser,[46] and also by Ryan and Foster[47] at the University of California.

The drug research highlights the dilemma of the general medical practitioner who is called upon to prescribe drugs for pain and other conditions by patients whom he hardly knows, and with no means at his disposal for assessing relevant personality factors. He may find in practice that a drug dosage which is suitably analgesic for some patients may seem to be quite useless for others, hence the ever-present medical suspicion that patients may be malingering, hypochondriacal and suffering from 'imaginary' pain.

The Systems of Eysenck and Petrie

It has been mentioned that the augmentation-reduction dimension of Petrie closely parallels the introversion-extraversion dimension of Eysenck. We have seen that in both experimental and clinical studies of pain it is the introverts and the augmenters who are the most susceptible, even though in certain circumstances it is the extraverts who complain most and make most demands for pain-relief. One has to go back to a paper Eysenck[48] published in 1955 to get the whole background of Petrie's work, and to see how it relates to earlier work by Köhler and Dinnerstein and Klein and Kretch with the brain-injured. In her influential book *Individuality in Pain and Suffering*,[49] the second edition of which was published in 1978, Petrie mentions these authors only in a footnote. The phenomenon of 'satiation' which Petrie mentions in her earlier published work is hardly mentioned in her book. Petrie records that people who react in one way to a test of their tactile experience are quite tolerant of pain, and people who react in another way are less tolerant. As others have found the same thing independently, it appears to be an established phenomenon, but the layman will find the whole matter rather mysterious and wonder *why* this should be so. If we turn to Eysenck, he offers an explanatory theory of the phenomenon which makes it more comprehensible.

What Petrie is testing with her wooden blocks of different sizes is a perceptual after-effect; that is, when we feel (or see) any object for a certain length of time it creates an impression in the relevant part of the brain, and temporary changes occur in the neural cells such that perceptual experiences of other objects in the immediate future will be altered by the after-effect. The after-effect of perceptual stimulation is held to be a neurological phenomenon of *satiation* of the relevant cells of the cerebral cortex of the brain. Eysenck holds that the essential difference between the extravert and the introvert, expressed in neurological terms, is that the former develops satiation (in Pavlov's terminology, 'inhibition') of the cerebral cortex more quickly, and retains it for a longer period than the introvert. Extraverts can therefore be expected to show after-effects from perceptual stimulation more readily, and the satiation will be manifest for longer. At the level of everyday observation we can observe that our more extraverted acquaintances will become bored with working at the same task for too long and seek relief in variety of stimulation. As has been pointed out, drugs like caffeine are cortical stimulants and hence introvert the personality temporarily, thereby lessening boredom and enabling us to concentrate on some task for longer. Drugs like alcohol have the opposite effect on the cerebral cortex; they extravert us and make us less capable of sustained concentration, which is what we want at parties when we wish to be more relaxed and enjoy ourselves.

Eysenck's 1955 paper, in which he referred to the work of Petrie and related it to that of earlier researchers, propounded the fundamentals of his theory of introversion-extraversion, and how it related to experiments with perceptual after-effects. The paper also reported a small study with twenty-eight psychiatric patients. They were allocated to the extraverted or introverted category mainly according to their diagnostic category (i.e. whether their disorders were of a hysteric/psychopathic or a dysthymic kind) but this categorization was supported by scores on the Rathymia scale of Guilford. (This was before the development of the MPI.) The patients were tested on the tactile perceptual apparatus, and it was found that the more extraverted group showed the greater after-effect. In Petrie's terms they were reducers.

In writing of 'introverts' and 'extraverts' it is natural to give the impression that there are two 'types' of personality: we give the same impression by referring to 'augmenters' and 'reducers'. This impression is misleading, for the systems of both Eysenck and Petrie are essentially *dimensional*; that is, it is recognized that only a few people are highly introverted or highly extraverted, and most of us are intermediate on the dimension, or as Petrie calls them, 'moderates'. However, for purposes of experiment either in the laboratory or in the clinical field, it is most useful to take contrasted groups from either end of the continuum.

Eysenck's 1955 paper has been cited as being of historic importance; he was later to develop his theory of personality considerably, and the form in which it is most relevant to the study of pain is that discussed in his book *The Biological Basis of Personality* (1967), which gives a wide review of clinical evidence, performance studies, drug research and even criminological studies. As mentioned earlier, Davidson and Bobey have referred to this work as bringing forward only the *supporting* evidence referring to a theory of individual difference in susceptibility to pain, but its interest lies in its relating pain experience to a wide and coherent theory of human behaviour. The basis of Eysenck's theory of personality, which derives from both Pavlov and Hull, involves consideration of the neurological events concerned in perception and learning.

Earlier in this chapter, the study of Lynn and Eysenck on pain tolerance was cited, and we may now refer back to it in more detail to try to understand why more extraverted people are more tolerant of pain. The initial paragraph of the paper expresses the essence of the theory well:

> It may be deduced from Eysenck's theory of personality . . . that pain tolerance should be *positively* related to extraversion (E) and *negatively* to neuroticism (N). Extraverted S[ubject]s are postulated to develop inhibition/satiation more quickly, and dissipate it more slowly; prolonged pain sensations should thus be inhibited more quickly and strongly in extraverts, leading to diminished pain sensations. Furthermore, as Beecher has pointed out, physiological pain sensations are always accompanied by the *apprehension of future pain*, which may be conceived of as a conditioned fear (anxiety) response which summates with the physiological pain. . . . Extraverts are posited to condition less well, and would therefore not develop this component of the total pain to the same extent as introverts. The prediction relating to N is perhaps less secure; it rests on the assumption that the strength of the autonomic reaction to pain stimulation would be likely to be related directly to N, which is conceived of in terms of autonomic lability.[50]

It may also be mentioned that in this study Lynn and Eysenck also used the Spiral After-effect Test, a visual test of doubtful validity, as well as the measure of pain, hoping to ascertain different degrees of susceptibility to cortical 'satiation', but the results they obtained with this measure were not statistically significant.

Later Related Evidence

Over the years the facts about individual differences in susceptibility to pain related to introversion-extraversion and to neuroticism, have come to be fairly widely accepted by those working in the clinical field and research, even by people who do not wholly accept Eysenck's theory of personality. The attempt by Petrie to link such research more closely with the study of stimulus deprivation has not been so successful, partly because of the many difficulties attending sensory deprivation experiments.

In later work on testing the augmentation-reduction tendency, the use of the tactile perception apparatus, which involves a very lengthy and tedious procedure, has been replaced by a more elegant technique, that of establishing differences in evoked potentials.

The study of evoked potentials began when it was found that the electrical activity of the brain in response to stimuli could be measured by putting electrodes on a subject's scalp, and connecting them to an electroencephalograph. The response to a stimulus can be measured in terms of latency (how long it takes the subject to respond) and amplitude (the magnitude of the response). The technique of successively increasing the strength of the stimulus (whether of light, sound or touch) produces a rising amplitude in the evoked potential up to a maximum, and then a decrease as 'satiation' develops. Individual differences in personality determine varying reactions to such procedures, and experiments with the tactile perceptual apparatus have shown that it measures the same phenomenon. A recent review of this experimental work is given by Barnes.[51]

The technique of testing individuals on the augmentation-reduction continuum by means of evoked potentials was developed in the 1960s by Silverman[52] and by Buchsbaum[53] in America. A great deal of work developed in the 1970s in Sweden, much of it under the direction of Von Knorring,[54] and it confirmed that different people's experience of pain was related to their status as augmenters or reducers as determined by the electrophysiological technique. The decade of the 1970s saw rapid and revolutionary development in pain research after the discovery of endorphins. Such research has been extended to the study of individual differences in the experience of pain, and of the augmentation-reduction and introversion-extraversion dimensions.

Before proceeding further it is as well to remind ourselves of the terminology which has been used by all those working in the same field as Petrie and Eysenck, and to recall that augmentation = introversion, and reduction = extraversion. *Absolute* equivalence is not claimed, as there are minor theoretical differences between the two systems; but there are strong reasons for getting the direction of the association clear before going on to consider the psychophysiological work which depends upon evoked potentials. First, a quote from Petrie:

> In another adult group of 38 persons in which the Maudsley Personality Inventory and perceptual reactance scores had been obtained, differences between reducers and augmenters in the expected direction were also found. The reducers provided significantly higher extraversion scores than did the augmenters (30.0 as against 23.8 –.01 probability level). There was again, in this group, no difference in the scores for neuroticism.[55]

This may be compared with a quote from Callaway, a specialist in evoked potentials:

> There seems a repeatable relationship between augmenting on the flash procedure and a general outgoing, distractible, maniclike, stimulus-seeking temperament. The augmenters score high on the Maudsley extraversion scale (Soskis and Shagass, 1974) and on the Zuckerman stimulus-seeking scale (Buchsbaum *et al.*, 1971; Zuckerman *et al.*, 1974). Patients with bi-polar affective disorders are augmenters, and lithium tends to convert them into reducers (Borge *et al.*, 1971; Buchsbaum *et al.*, 1971).[56]

It is perfectly clear that the electrophysiologists and those following their methods first accepted the work of Petrie (to whom they routinely give credit) and then *stood her terminology upside-down.* For them, augmentation = reduction, and reduction = augmentation. It is as simple as that. Once one has accepted this complete inversion of terms, all their work is comprehensible and in accord with the twenty years of antecedent research, including the established relations with toleration of pain and with extraversion. Justification for this complete reversal of terminology is not accepted by the present writer. It is possible that the confusion that it has caused is partly responsible for the fact that the electrophysiological research is now largely ignored by an influential section of those engaged in pain research, a neglect which seems highly regrettable in view of its potential promise. A number of researchers are under the impression that the *facts* about augmentation-reduction are very contradictory; but this is not the case.

In Barnes'[57] substantial review of the literature on augmentation-reduction, he does indeed call attention to the strange inversion of terminology by the electrophysiologists, but he can give no adequate explanation for it. He does, however, make the useful point that we may make a distinction between 'state' and 'trait' with regard to the augmentation-reduction. An individual may have a constitutional tendency to augment; that is his tendency by trait. In certain circumstances, perhaps because of this pronounced trait, he may be forced into a reaction of extreme reduction, e.g. by the consumption of alcohol or, as Petrie has suggested, by pathological conditions such as schizophrenic illness. It should be noted that much of the work of the electrophysiologists, including that carried out in Sweden, has been done with psychiatric populations. But this does not entirely clear up the confusion and one feels that it is up to those who have reversed the terminology to make special efforts to do so.

Eysenck has written as follows about the confusion of terminology:

In my early work on figural aftereffects, and in Petrie's adaptation of it, we were concerned with input into the nervous system, and it makes sense to say that the introvert, because of his high arousal level, augments incoming sensations, while the extravert, because of his low arousal, reduces them. Buchsbaum and his colleagues, however, are concerned with output, and thus invoke Pavlov's law of transmarginal inhibition. This states that with increasing input, an optimal point will be reached beyond which output does not increase, but decrease. Buchsbaum is concerned with what happens beyond this point, and clearly therefore increasing sensations, as shown by Petrie's augmenters, will be evidenced in terms of decreasing output, i.e. reduction. Buchsbaum has fastened on to this reduction, and consequently calls Petrie's augmenters (input) reducers (output).[58]

Many people will find the position profoundly unsatisfactory when researchers use contrary terminology, and wonder whether their efforts will further our understanding of individual differences in susceptibility to pain. We must take the research field as we find it, however, and hope that in the course of time the anomalies will be sorted out. What follows is reported because of its considerable intrinsic interest, and because it indicates the probable lines of an important section of pain research for the future.

Some Directions for Future Research

In conditions of chronic pain, it is likely that the activity of the endorphin-secreting system is altered, as has been shown by Almay,[59] Sjölund[60] and their colleagues, and that individual differences in augmentation-reduction relate to this system. Research on endorphins was initially hampered by the difficulty of assessing the quantity present in the neural tissue at any time. Originally the presence of endorphins was inferred from the results of injecting substances such as naloxone which block their action, as described in the previous chapter. Buchsbaum et al.[61] showed that injection of naloxone would alter both pain perception and evoked potentials.

Important among the studies relating levels of endorphins to differences in reaction to the evoked potential technique, is that of Von Knorring et al.[62] Forty-five patients admitted to hospital with conditions of chronic pain had their level of endorphins in the cerebrospinal fluid assessed by a technique which had recently been perfected. The status of each patient on the augmentation-reduction dimension was determined by the evoked potential technique, and it was found that those with a greater tendency to augment stimuli (i.e. the amplitude of response *increases* when stimulus intensity increases) were found to have significantly lower levels of endorphins than patients whose response was to reduce stimuli (i.e. the amplitude of response *decreases* when stimulus intensity increases). This does not imply a causative relationship; we do not know whether the level of endorphins follows from the habitual type of perceptual reactance, or vice versa.

This study is complemented by that of Johansson et al.,[63] who administered several personality questionnaires to forty chronic pain patients in Sweden. They used Swedish translations of the Zuckerman Sensation Seeking Scale (SSS), which has good measures of extraversion labelled 'Thrill-seeking, Experience-seeking, Disinhibition and Boredom-Susceptibility', and the Eysenck Personality Inventory (EPI). A third personality test (in Swedish) was also used, the Cesarek Marke Personality Scheme (CMPS) which relates to the old personality scheme of Murray,[64] and tests the strength of eleven allegedly basic 'needs'. (It may be remarked, in passing, that the weakness of personality tests like the CMPS, which have a great number of scales, is that what you lose on the swings you are likely to gain on the roundabouts by sheer chance, so to speak; there is an increased probability that entirely fortuitous associations will show up.)

A sample of cerebrospinal fluid was taken from each patient, and the concentration of endorphins was assessed by the same method Von Knorring had used. For purposes of comparison, thirty healthy subjects also completed the personality tests, but they did not have their endorphin levels assessed.

Comparing the personality scores of the pain patients with those of the healthy subjects, it was found that the former were more introverted and more neurotic, a finding that accords with the great majority of research studies conducted over the past thirty years. Specifically, the scores on the SSS were significantly lower for the pain patients, but scores on the EPI, although in the expected direction, were not significantly different statistically. Three of the eleven CMPSs showed some significant relationship, the pain patients showing more 'guilt feelings' and need for 'order', and less 'autonomy', findings which might apply to any group of chronic patients.

Turning to the relationship between endorphin levels and personality scores in the patient group, the five scales of the SSS indicated that those with a higher degree of extraversion had a lower level of concentration of endorphins in the cerebrospinal fluid. The EPI neuroticism scores indicated that the lower the level of endorphins, the lower the level of neuroticism. In this study therefore, the 'neurotic introvert' type among pain patients was found to have a higher concentration of endorphins.

These two studies are mentioned as examples of the sort of research that is proceeding in Sweden, but they do not do full justice to the amount and range of the Swedish research relating endorphin levels to personality variables and individual differences in experience of and susceptibility to pain. It has already been mentioned that, at the time of writing, such research has been largely ignored by an influential section of pain researchers in other countries, although reports of it are now appearing in the international journal *Pain* and other widely-read journals. The confusion of terms over the concept of augmenting and reducing, to which attention has been drawn here, may be related to this lack of cohesion in research, and it is to be hoped that it will soon be resolved.

Conclusion

Cronbach[65] has referred to 'The two disciplines of scientific psychology'. Broadly, he makes a distinction between the researchers and theory-builders who consider individual differences in behaviour and experience as the prime object of study whereby the causative mechanisms of phenomena may be elucidated, and a second group who regard such individual differences merely as a nuisance that complicates research and is best ignored or discounted in studying general principles. This division exists in pain research. As was mentioned at the beginning of this chapter, each of us realizes early in our own experience that there are significant individual differences in susceptibility to pain: in trying to come to grips with this problem, scientific research has developed from the early efforts with paper-and-pencil tests and relatively crude procedures involving wooden blocks, to more sophisticated measurements with electrophysiological apparatus and assays of endorphin levels. The later methods are not more 'scientific', since science is a matter of method and reasoning rather than technological sophistication, but the later methods continue to show promise in expanding our understanding of the mechanisms underlying the experience of pain, and of the methods we may use to control it.

REFERENCES

1 W. E. Fordyce, *Behavioral Methods for Chronic Pain and Illness*, St Louis: Mosleys, 1978.

2 E. J. Shoben and L. Borland, 'An empirical study of the etiology of dental fears', *Journal of Clinical Psychology*, 1954, 10, pp. 171–4.

3 R. Johnson and D. C. Baldwin, 'Relationship of maternal anxiety to the behaviour of young children undergoing dental extraction', *Journal of Dental Research*, 1968, 47, pp. 801–5.

4 M. Zborowski, 'Cultural components in responses to pain', *Journal of Social Issues*, 1952, 8, pp. 16–30.

5 C. D. Spielberger, R. L. Gorsuch and R. E. Luskine, *Manual of the State-Trait Anxiety Inventory*, Palo Alto, Calif.: Consulting Psychologists Press, 1970.

6 N. L. Corah, 'Development of a dental anxiety scale', *Journal of Dental Research*, 1969, 48, pp. 596–601.

7 M. Weisenberg, M. L. Kreindler, R. Schachat and J. Werboff, 'Pain: anxiety and attitudes in black, white and Puerto Rican patients', *Journal of Psychosomatic Medicine*, 1975, 37, pp. 123–35.

8 B. Tursky and R. A. Sternbach, 'Further physiological correlates of ethnic differences in response to shock', *Psychophysiology*, 1967, 4, pp. 67–74.

9 M. Zborowski, *People in Pain*, San Francisco: Jossey Bass, 1969.

10 K. M. Woodrow, G. D. Friedman, A. B. Siegelaub and M. F. Collen, 'Pain differences according to age, sex and race', *Psychosomatic Medicine*, 1972, 34, pp. 548–56.

11 W. E. Lambert, W. E. Bibman and E. G. Poser, 'The effect of increased salience of a membership group on pain tolerance', *Journal of Personality*, 1960, 38, pp. 350–9.

12 R. Lynn and H. J. Eysenck, 'Tolerance for pain, extraversion and neuroticism', *Perceptual and Motor Skills*, 1961, 12, pp. 161–2.

13 D. Haslam, 'Individual differences in pain threshold and level of arousal', *British Journal of Psychology*, 1967, 58, pp. 139–42.

14 F. M. Levine, B. Tursky and D. C. Nichols, 'Tolerance for pain, extraversion and neuroticism: failure to replicate results', *Perceptual and Motor Skills*, 1966, 23, pp. 847–50.

15 P. O. Davidson and M. J. Bobey, 'Repressor-Sensitizer differences on repeated exposures to pain', *Perceptual and Motor Skills*, 1970, 31, pp. 711–14.

16 J. E. Martin and J. Inglis, 'Pain tolerance and narcotic addiction', *British Journal of Social and Clinical Psychology*, 1965, 4, pp. 224-9.

17 P. O. Davidson and M. J. Bobey, op. cit.

18 P. O. Davidson and C. E. A. McDougall, 'Personality and pain tolerance measures', *Perceptual and Motor Skills*, 1969, 28, pp. 787-90.

19 H. J. Eysenck, *The Biological Basis of Personality*, Springfield, Ill.: C. C. Thomas, 1967.

20 M. R. Bond and I. B. Pearson, 'Psychological aspects of pain in women with advanced cancer of the cervix', *Journal of Psychosomatic Research*, 1969, 13, pp. 13-19.

21 A. Petrie, *Individuality in Pain and Suffering*, 2nd Edition, Chicago: University of Chicago Press, 1978.

22 H. Merskey, 'Personality traits of psychiatric patients with pain', *Journal of Psychosomatic Research*, 1972, 16, pp. 163-6.

23 A. Petrie, op. cit., p. 61.

24 R. A. Sternbach, *Pain Patients: Traits and Treatment*, op. cit.

25 L. F. Pilling, T. F. Brannick and W. M. Swenson, 'Psychological characteristics of psychiatric patients having pain as a presenting symptom', *Canadian Medical Association Journal*, 1967, 97, pp. 387-94.

26 K. Jamison, M. T. Ferrer-Brechner, V. L. Brechner and C. P. McCreary, 'Correlations of personality profile with pain syndrome', in J. J. Bonica and D. Albe-Fessard (eds), *Advances in Pain Research and Therapy*, op. cit.

27 R. A. Sternbach, op. cit.

28 See R. Adler, 'The differentiation of organic and psychogenic pain', *Pain*, 1981, 10, pp. 249-52.

29 R. Melzack, 'Psychological concepts and methods for the control of pain', in J. J. Bonica (ed.), *Advances in Neurology*, op. cit., p. 277.

30 A. Taub, 'Symposium discussion', ibid., p. 612.

31 F. J. Spear, 'Pain in psychiatric patients', *Journal of Psychosomatic Research*, 1967, 11, pp. 187-93.

32 A. Petrie, *Personality and the Frontal Lobes*, London: Routledge & Kegan Paul, 1952.

33 W. Freeman and J. W. Watts, *Psychosurgery in the Treatment of Mental Disorders and Intractable Pain*, op. cit.

34 A. Petrie, *Individuality in Pain and Suffering*, op. cit., p. 17.

35 L. Von Knorring, *The Experience of Pain in Patients with Depressive Disorders*, Umeå: University Medical Dissertations, 1975.

36 G. S. Klein and D. Krech, 'Cortical conductivity in the brain-injured', *Journal of Personality*, 1952, 21, pp. 118-48.

37 For a full description of the testing apparatus see A. Petrie, *Individual Differences in Pain and Suffering*, op. cit., Appendix A.

38 W. H. Bexton, W. Heron and T. H. Scott, 'Effects of decreased variation in sensory environment', *Canadian Journal of Psychology*, 1954, 8, pp. 70-6.

39 A. Petrie, W. Collins and P. Solomon, 'Pain sensitivity, sensory deprivation and susceptibility to satiation', *Science*, 1958, 128, pp. 1431-3.

40 J. P. Zubeck (ed.), *Sensory Deprivation: Fifteen Years of Research*, New York: Appleton-Century-Crofts, 1969.

41 J. G. Minard, 'Prediction of sensory deprivation tolerance and post-session depression from tasks involving stimulus inspection', Paper read at Eastern Psychology Association, New York, 1966.

42 M. Zuckerman, 'Variables affecting deprivation results', in J. P. Zubeck (ed.), *Sensory Deprivation*, op. cit., p. 80.

43 A. Petrie, *Individuality in Pain and Suffering*, op. cit., p. 39.

44 P. B. Bradley, 'The central action of certain drugs in relation to the reticular formation of the brain', in H. H. Jasper (ed.), *Reticular Formation of the Brain*, Edinburgh: Churchill, 1957.

45 A. Petrie, *Individuality in Pain and Suffering*, op. cit. p. 61.

46 E. G. Poser, 'Figural after-effect as a personality correlate', in *Proceedings of 16th International Congress of Psychology*, Amsterdam: N. Holland Publishing Co., 1960.

47 E. D. Ryan and R. Foster, 'Athletic participation and perceptual augmentation and reduction', *Journal of Personality and Social Psychology*, 1967, 6, pp. 472-6.

48 H. J. Eysenck 'Cortical inhibition, figural aftereffect and theory of personality', *Journal of Abnormal and Social Psychology*, 1955, 51, pp. 94-106.

49 A. Petrie, *Individuality in Pain and Suffering*, op. cit.

50 R. Lynn and H. J. Eysenck, 'Tolerance for pain, extraversion and neuroticism', op. cit.

51 G. E. Barnes, 'Individual differences in perceptual reactance: A review of the stimulus intensity modulation individual difference dimension', *Canadian Psychological Review*, 1976, 17, pp. 29-52.

52 J. Silverman, 'Perceptual control of stimulus intensity in paranoid and non-paranoid schizophrenia', *Journal of Nervous and Mental Diseases*, 1964, 139, pp. 545-9.

53 M. S. Buchsbaum and J. Silverman, 'Stimulus intensity control and the control of evoked response', *Psychosomatic Medicine*, 1968, 30, pp. 12-22.

54 L. Von Knorring, *The Experience of Pain in Patients with Depressive Disorders*, Umeä: University of Umeä, 1975.

55 A. Petrie, *Individuality in Pain and Suffering*, op. cit., p. 36.

56 E. Callaway, *Brain Electrical Potentials and Individual Psychological Differences*, New York: Grune & Stratton, 1975.

57 G. E. Barnes, 'Individual differences in perceptual reactance', op. cit.

58 H. J. Eysenck, Personal communication dated 22 June, 1981.

59 B. G. L. Almay, F. Johansson, L. Von Knorring, L. Terenius and A. Wahlström, 'Endorphins in chronic pain: I Differences in CSF endorphin levels between organic and psychogenic pain syndromes', *Pain*, 1978, 5, pp 153-62.

60 B. Sjölund, L. Terenius and M. Eriksson, 'Increased cerebro-spinal fluid levels after electroacupuncture', *Acta Physiologica Scandinavia*, 1977, 100, pp. 382-4.

61 M. S. Buchsbaum, G. C. Davis and W. E. Bunney, 'Naloxone alters pain perception and somatosensory evoked potentials in normal subjects,' *Nature*, 1977, 270, pp. 620-1.

62 L. Von Knorring, B. G. L. Almay, F. Johansson and L. Terenius, 'Endorphins in CSF of chronic pain patients, in relation to augmenting-reducing response in visual average evoked response', *Neuropsychobiology*, 1979, 5, pp. 322-6.

63 F. Johansson, B. G. L. Almay, L. Von Knorring, L. Terenius and M. Åström, 'Personality traits in chronic pain patients related to endorphin levels in cerebrospinal fluid', *Psychiatry Research*, 1979, 1, pp. 231-9.

64 H. A. Murray, *Explorations of Personality*, New York: Oxford University Press, 1938.

65 L. J. Cronbach, 'The two disciplines in scientific psychology', *American Psychologist*, 1957, 12, pp. 671-84.

7

THE NATURE AND TREATMENT
OF CHRONIC PAIN

The Problem

Pain that is immediate and transient is beneficent and of biological advantage, teaching all animals to avoid injury and to live healthily. Earlier chapters have related the history of how mankind has learnt to deal with the pain of accidental injuries, and of that incidental to surgery willingly undergone. Acute pain is a good physician and advises us when matters are going wrong, but chronic pain serves no such useful function. Because of the curious neurological and psychological make-up of the animal organism, pain can persist with evil intensity long after an organic lesion has healed. Earlier, we discussed the case of phantom limb pain, where the pain is felt to exist in a limb which is no longer present. Physicians have learnt not to insist that a patient is insane, 'imagining' or malingering when he declares that he has chronic pain in his non-existent foot, but the sufferer from a similar phantom pain is sometimes less successful in convincing the physician of the reality of his chronic pain when it relates to a part of the body which is still present, and on physical examination shows no apparent pathology. Chronic pain bears the same relationship to acute, transient pain, that neurotic phobias bear to to the healthy fear mechanisms which protect us in conditions of danger. Both chronic pain and neurotic phobias can be learned, and once learned they are difficult to remove.

Chronic pain commonly causes severe physical, emotional and social stresses in the sufferer. Although not drastically unwell or physically disabled, he may be severely crippled by the experience of constant pain and an unhappy burden to his family. It is difficult to be a patient invalid when one is in pain, and it is difficult to bear with people who have nothing obviously wrong with them but who constantly complain about their private experience of pain. Again, one is reminded of the neurotic who appears to be healthy but who constantly complains that life is hell.

We can all emphathize with the experience of acute pain, but chronic pain has a quality which is fundamentally different. When pain becomes chronic, the autonomic reflexes which we regard as characteristic of pain may disappear; physical degeneration may set in due to loss of appetite and disturbed feeding habits, to habitual loss of sleep, and to the very drugs that the physician prescribes to overcome the pain. Many 'pain patients', as they are called, also suffer from the neurological damage that surgeons have inflicted in well-meant but vain efforts to sever the neural pathways that were supposed to carry the messages of pain. The anxiety associated with acute pain becomes replaced by the long-term reactive depression of the chronic sufferer, and here a behavioural vicious circle may set in, for the more the patient withdraws from life the greater will be his pain experience and his hypochondriacal habits.

Just as in the mid nineteenth century medical science was in a turmoil over the problem of acute pain, a turmoil characterized by many violent and absurd controversies, so in the late twentieth century we are struggling with the problems of chronic pain. Furthermore, science has broadened so that today the problem is one that concerns many specialisms other than medicine and surgery. Psychologists, pharmacologists, sociologists, physiologists, psychiatrists and other specialists are involved, each with their useful contribution, and of course their bid for the power and prestige of their discipline. That the orthodox practitioners of therapeutic science have been hitherto rather unsuccessful in adequately treating the problems of chronic pain, is highlighted by the fact that many long-term sufferers, after they have been through the hands of physicians, surgeons and other genuine professionals, turn in desperation to faith-healers, astrologers, quack hypnotists, herbalists, self-taught acupuncturists and purveyors of black boxes. Because of the curious psychological nature of chronic pain, the strange régime proposed by some mountebank may succeed in relieving pain when methods based on science have failed. Or so one hears: hard evidence about such occurrences is difficult to come by.

How is it that in this advanced and technical age bio-medical science has made so little headway in the understanding and treatment of chronic pain? According to Bonica, one of the reasons is that scientists have used the evidence obtained from the study of acute pain, and applied it to the problems of chronic pain without being fully aware that the latter is 'a totally different phenomenon'.[1] He explains the general incompetence of the medical profession adequately to deal with chronic pain in terms of the inappropriate teaching in medical schools.

Added to this confusion is the relative lack of communication between the different disciplines involved. One has to consult a very wide spectrum of scientific journals, which are seldom all available in any one university library, to collate the different approaches to chronic pain taken by the various specialisms. The wretched patient who suffers from this condition must, if his GP sends him to a specialist, take pot luck as to whatever specialists are available in his area. He may end up with an anaesthesiologist who proposes to inject nerve blocks into him, a dynamic psychiatrist who wants to investigate his Oedipus complex, or a neurosurgeon who wants to sever some of his nerves or coagulate areas of his brain.

The average GP, bombarded as he is with a stream of literature emanating from the drug manufacturers, is likely to be strongly biased towards treating chronic pain with drugs. He is well aware of the twin problems of *tolerance* (when the same dosage no longer has any effect) and *physical dependence* (illness or craving if the drug is withdrawn), but he knows no other way of responding to his patients' complaints of pain. It will take a little while before the considerable research findings of the last decade make their impact on the overworked GP.

Identifying the 1970s as the truly fruitful decade for the application of new discoveries in the treatment of pain is not to disparage the work of earlier times which built up to a cumulative breakthrough in the application of theory to practice. There has been a great increase in the collaboration between various scientists and clinicians, so that the old distinction between medical and non-medical workers hardly applies. The International Association for the Study of Pain has been founded, and held its first World Congress in Florence in 1975, a congress attended by more than a thousand scientists, physicians and other health professionals. Some idea of the scope of the specialisms represented will be gained by seeing their variety as set out in Appendix 1 at the end of this book.

Back-Ache

Of all the causes of pain to which mankind, and particularly womankind, is subject, back-ache is one of the most common and distressful. It is a source of both direct and indirect suffering, and because of its consequences, there builds up a whole syndrome of restrictions on social and physical activities which creates a vicious circle of mounting, chronic pain. When an injured back has recovered, or partly recovered, the actual pains may be so slight that they would normally be disregarded as a minor nuisance by a person immersed in the preoccupations of work, hobbies, social activities, family life and general pleasures, but when all these become restricted, this little occasional pain becomes magnified to a fantastic degree and may dominate life. It becomes no longer a 'little' and 'occasional' pain, but a really bad state of pain which nags at the sufferer night and day.

Readers who have appreciated the exposition of the nature of pain put forward in this book, will have no difficulty in understanding how a little pain may become transmuted into a really severe pain, not by any change in the physical condition which is producing it, but by the drastic restriction of the normal pleasures of everyday life. It is as though the energy which should be discharged in constructive activity and pleasure becomes dammed up and converted into pain. This rather picturesque way of thinking of potential pleasure becoming expressed as pain is, of course, at the basis of much psychoanalytic thinking. Freud's theorizing about the economy of the libido became very complex indeed in his later writings,[2] but in simple terms the theory envisages energy which should normally be directed and discharged in creative and satisfying channels becoming converted into anxiety, or in certain cases, into pain.

In his earlier works Freud wrote extensively of 'conversion symptoms', that is, symptoms depending on the conversion of the libido in the manner described above. Discussing his patient Elizabeth von R., he wrote, 'She repressed her erotic idea from consciousness and transformed the amount of its affect into physical pain.'[3] The normal sufferer from a very real organic lesion in the back may object to the comparison of his condition with a hysterical conversion symptom, but the purpose here is not to imply that his is a 'hysterical' rather than a 'real' pain. I would certainly not go the whole way with the Freudians in theorizing about pain. Nevertheless, Freud fully realized that organic conditions might underlie the maintenance of the conversion of dammed-up affect into pain.

Merskey and Spear[4] have summarized Freud's early thinking about the way in which pain becomes very greatly magnified by the restriction of channels of normal expression of energy, and they list seven points, only four of which they regard as valid in the light of later research. The present author would not go as far as Merskey and Spear, particularly with regard to the Freudian belief that pain generally has a symbolic meaning, a contention which appears to lack any empirical proof or possibility of proof. All that seems clear is that unexpressed 'nervous energy', to use a useful layman's term, is often experienced as pain when there is an existing organic substratum, or perhaps more rarely, when there *was* originally a pain-producing lesion which is now substantially healed.

The sufferer from back-pain is very vulnerable to this unfortunate conversion mechanism because of the many restrictions on activity caused by this condition, and paradoxically the strong, vigorous person accustomed to physical activity is in a rather worse plight than then the less vigorous type of person.

Back-pain may also constrain the sufferer's sex life. The man or woman who is accustomed to regular and satisfying sex relations will find them drastically disrupted by an injury to the lower back because the type of pelvic movements which normally take place in copulation now cause pain. If the man is the back sufferer, he may find that his normal movements in the sex act are so painful that he is unable to proceed, bringing frustration to himself and his partner. The woman's pelvic movements, if she is the sufferer, may be equally painful; she becomes inhibited herself and the knowledge of her discomfort restrains her partner.

The extent to which one can alter established patterns of sexual intercourse depends upon one's individual constitution. Nevertheless, it is important that sufferers from back-pain who have previously enjoyed a full sex life should not abandon sexual relations on account of their pain. If sexual tension and energy is allowed to build up, it is likely to be experienced as a magnification of the pain already suffered. The sufferer and his partner are advised to experiment with different techniques until they find one (or more) that is mutually satisfying. There are available a number of useful publications dealing with sexual techniques, including these suitable for the disabled, and giving advice which will help in the recognition of the nature of the problem and how to solve it.[5]

Learning and Unlearning Pain

It is very important that the sufferer from back-ache should restrict his or her life as little as possible. Obviously, if previous to the injury football or some other strenuous sport was played, he cannot continue when physically incommoded, but he should beware of merely 'resting' in the time which he used to devote to the sport. Indeed, he should avoid rewarding himself for pains in the back by too much comfort, a nice drink, sympathetic attention from family and friends, and any more indulgence in the fleshpots than had been his previous habit. Such indulgence is fine – but not as a *reward* for pain, or the pain will increase in frequency and severity.

This is an extremely difficult matter to understand: on the one hand we are advocating that the true antagonist of pain is pleasure, and on the other hand issuing a warning that pleasure may be an insidious danger. A full understanding of the nature of operant conditioning needs to be achieved before it will be appreciated how pleasure, treated as a *reward* for pain, can actually increase the sum total of pain.

The prescription that indulgence should be withheld from the sufferer sounds harsh, but if the sufferer understands the relevant mechanisms it is he himself who will initiate the discipline.

Operant conditioning refers to the process whereby a response becomes more frequent if it is immediately rewarded. In this process the temporal relationship between the response and the reward is crucial. Originating with the work of Skinner[6] many years ago, research has shown that not only will a particular random movement come to be repeated more frequently if it is immediately rewarded (i.e. the animal or person receives something pleasant like a food reward, praise or the immediate interruption of something unpleasant), but also that physiological reactions such as an increase in heartbeat or the dilation of blood-vessels in a particular part can be made to occur by this conditioning procedure.[7] Thus, not only is habitual behaviour, including many actions which take place automatically without conscious intention, governed by its immediate consequences, but many sensory experiences are similarly determined.

Originally, Skinner made a distinction between two kinds of responses, which he called 'respondents' and 'operants'. Respondents are reactions to antecedent stimuli; in the classical conditioning of Pavlov, the salivation of a dog is the respondent to the presentation of meat, and this respondent can become attached to the antecedent stimulus of the sound of a bell. On the other hand, operants are actions which are more under deliberate control, but their occurrence may be encouraged by frequent reward, the reward being presented immediately after the action. Thus in animal experimentation, if every time a pigeon stretched its left wing a food reward appeared, the bird would develop the habit of frequently making that movement. This acquired habit will persist after it is established if it is occasionally rewarded, but if the rewards cease altogether it will become less and less frequent, until eventually it ceases altogether, except as an occasional and random movement as before.

Normally we think of our actions as occurring in response to some antecedent stimulus, including a predetermined intention on our part, but operants are a curious class of behaviours which occur habitually without our deliberately intending them. The original distinction that was made between respondents and operants has been somewhat broken down by the work that has been done by Neal Miller and his associates on conditioning physiological responses. As mentioned above, many sensory experiences and glandular responses have been shown to be subject to operant conditioning.[8]

The relevance of this to conditions of chronic pain is that the whole life of the chronic sufferer becomes hemmed around by various syndromes of experience and behaviour which are known as 'pain behaviour', and this includes the subjective suffering. Fordyce expresses the position thus:

> The clinician may observe various autonomic manifestations of pain. Mainly, however, the data he uses are based on auditory and visual information from the patient. The patient may moan, grimace, or move in a guarded fashion. He may talk about his pain. He may report or be observed to display functional impairment from his pain; for example, spending a great deal of time in bed because it hurts too much to move. All of those events are operants. As such, they are subject to influence by consequences. It is easy to underestimate the significance of that statement.[9]

Fordyce goes on to develop the view that it is therefore scientifically sound to consider the possibility that a sufferer's pain may have come under the control of learning factors, such factors being environmental consequences. If the chronic patient has come under such control there is no need to postulate the existence of any kind of underlying pathology which is currently responsible for his pain behaviour. He has learned pain behaviour by the process of operant conditioning, just as another type of sufferer may have learned a totally irrational phobia which dominates his life.

In saying that there may be no underlying pathology which is currently responsible for his pain behaviour, it is perhaps more realistic to suggest that although some small pathology is probably present, it is giving rise to far, far more pain than it should if we view the condition in neurological terms. But if the pain behaviour has been learned, then theoretically it can be unlearned by appropriate treatment, and this holds a ray of hope for the sufferer.

If we accept the theory of operant conditioning, then behaviour is governed by its consequences, and hence is being maintained by the 'rewards' it receives. Here we must stress that the term 'rewards' is being used entirely technically, for anyone suffering from a pain condition will legitimately and forcefully point out that he would willingly forgo any such 'rewards' if he could be free of his pain, normally active and enjoying life. Similarly, the sufferer from a crippling phobia which dominates his life would willingly forgo the 'rewards' which maintain his pattern of fear and withdrawal, but, without help, is unable to break out of the habit which has ensnared him. To eliminate a pattern of behaviour that has been acquired through the mechanisms of operant conditioning, two alternative techniques have been shown to be effective experimentally. The first is to stop supplying the accustomed 'reward': thus if a laboratory pigeon has acquired the habit of repeatedly stretching its left wing because it is under the control of a carefully planned schedule of the delivery of peas at the right moment, total cessation of the supply of peas will result in extinction of the habit. The second technique that will break the habit is to decide on some behavioural response which is *incompatible* with wing-stretching and carefully to cultivate it by a planned schedule of 'reward'.

It is a far cry from the experimental animal laboratory to the problems of the pain patient in hospital or living at home. However, as the proof of the pudding is in the eating, so the usefulness of a theory is to be judged by the actual results of its application in clinical practice. Before going on to cite actual clinical work, we may pursue the theory a little further. Fordyce refers to 'rewards' as 'reinforcers', and discusses the application of the two techniques for eliminating an unwanted habit in the context of hospitalized pain patients. He writes:

> If, for example, in the context of pain a patient were lying down more than was desirable, one might try to decrease time in bed by withdrawing positive reinforcers to such behaviour. Or, alternatively, one might attach effective positive reinforcers to incompatible behaviour such as walking.[10]

All this seems merely common sense, and some people may wonder what is served by parading common sense in the guise of science. But here we may quote Thomas Huxley who stated that 'Science is nothing but trained and organized common sense': the trouble about common sense as it is usually applied is that it is neither trained nor organized, and leads the lay person to such erroneous conclusions that a patient either has a 'real' pain reflecting an active organic injury, or that he is shamming. Common sense does not lead readily to an understanding of how not only the observable habits of the pain patient are learned, but also the subjective experience of pain, and, what is more to the point, how both can be unlearned. A common-sense pep talk to a patient who lies in bed too much may do more harm than good, and merely convince him that he has an unsympathetic and ignorant nurse. To withdraw the subtle positive reinforcers of too much bed-rest, requires a sensitive understanding of just what is 'rewarding' for that particular patient. Similarly, it is not easy to discover the effective positive reinforcers to incompatible behaviour such as walking.

Earlier, reference was made to a certain similarity between the chronic pain patient and the person who suffers from a severe phobia. In both cases there is some element of learning; in the former the learning is on the basis of an originally severe and partly persistent organic lesion, and in the latter the basis is an entirely rational fear mechanism, possibly with an 'instinctual' component which is innate.[11] It is thought that in phobic conditions the patient has been subjected to avoidance conditioning, that is, when he first experienced a slight fear for a certain class of objects (e.g. cats) or situations (e.g. being shut in a closed place) he learned a number of negative acts to avoid coming into contact with the fear-producing thing or situation. Through the mechanisms of operant conditioning, reduction of anxiety being the 'reward', he learns an ever-growing repertoire of negative habits, and so the established cat-phobic or claustrophobic, although he may never have encountered a cat at close quarters for many years, or been shut in an enclosed place, may have his behaviour severely circumscribed by a series of elaborate fear-avoidance rituals of which he is deeply ashamed yet is helpless to resist.[12] What fear is to the one type of patient, pain is to the other. Conditioning in avoidance learning teaches the pain patient a number of incommoding habits which persist because of the feared consequence of breaking these habits. He himself may not be entirely aware of these habits; for instance, he may hold himself in an odd posture, tensing certain muscle groups in a manner which leads to fatigue, and walking in a peculiar way, not because a normal posture and gait would hurt, but because this conditioned avoidance behaviour has become part of his normal behaviour repertoire. Similarly, his habits of resting, avoiding certain normal occupations, and his pill-swallowing, may be governed more by the operant avoidance conditioning than by the somatically generated pain which would follow from the non-observance of these habits.

The habit of pill-swallowing deserves especial mention because of all we now know about the power of placebos to inhibit pain. As discussed elsewhere in this book, it has been found that swallowing, or receiving by injection, totally inert substances can have such a powerful effect on the experience of pain that, to quote Evans, 'a placebo is about half as effective as morphine in relieving pain'.[13] The placebo effect exemplifies the mechanism of operant conditioning. We eat food because eating behaviour is governed by the consequences of a pleasant taste, a full stomach and a sensation of well-being. Similarly, we learn that the swallowing of pills has the desired effect of allaying pain. Having swallowed the pills, the pain will begin to remit long before the drug has time to exert its analgesic effect. But once the chronic pain patient becomes accustomed to swallowing a certain quantity of pills every day of his life (even when he has habituated to the action of the drug so thoroughly that he might as well be swallowing sugar pills), if he omits to take some or all of his pills a *negative* placebo effect will occur, and he will experience pain. How, then, do we get our drug addict to relinquish some or all of his daily diet of pills, which, although they may have ceased to have much pharmacological effect relative to his pain experience, certainly place a strain on his body's whole metabolism?

With the drug-addicted patient the problem is complicated by the fact that swallowing pills tends to be contingent on experiencing pain. Superficially, this appears to be only common sense, but it creates the situation that pain is *rewarded* by pills. In a hospital setting there may also be an additional reward, because the pill-swallowing is accompanied by attention from a nurse. Such attention is a very powerful 'reward' and consequently reinforces some aspects of pain behaviour.

One approach to the drug problem which has been tried at the Department of Rehabilitation Medicine at the University of Washington is to abandon the 'cafeteria system' of drug administration, and – having first carefully assessed each patient's daily drug intake – to combine all the drugs in a single capsule.[14] The capsule is then given on a *time-contingent* rather than a *pain-contingent* basis. Thus the experience of pain is not an operant which is 'rewarded' (and thereby maintained) by pain-contingent pills. At first the patient gets the same drug level as before, but a careful record is kept of level of reported pain at stated intervals, the amount of sleep he gets, his daily activity level and all such relevant matters. The strength of the pharmacological agents within the capsule can be cautiously reduced or altered without this coming to the attention of the patient, although he is not, of course, kept in ignorance of the fact that it is the general intention to modify the drug dosage. Keeping the patient in ignorance of alterations of the dosage within the capsule is no insult to his intelligence; it merely reflects the fact that it is quite impossible *not* to be influenced by the knowledge that one has taken more or less of a drug. Most researchers studying the effects of drugs deliberately keep themselves in ignorance of which patients are receiving the drug, and which the placebo, whilst the experimental trial is in progress, because they know very well that they would be influenced in their judgements by such knowledge, hence the methodology of the double-blind trial.[15]

The second factor which is given special attention in contingency management of chronic pain patients, is rest. Rest is naturally a very important 'reward' for pain: typically the patient exercises or works until pain comes on, then he rests. This seems a sensible procedure, but if rest is made pain-contingent then the same objections apply as with making pill-swallowing the 'reward' for pain. The régime that is applied at the Washington rehabilitation department is first to establish the tolerance level of activity for a patient, i.e. the amount of activity in which he can safely engage without pain coming on. He is then set a quota of activity which, initially, is *less* than his tolerance level, and a set scheme of rest periods. Thus rest is a 'reward' contingent upon exercise and not upon pain. This quota is then very gradually increased, with careful monitoring of all the other records of the patient's progress, and it is found in practice that the activity of the patient can generally be increased very substantially without him suffering pain. This treatment is similar in many ways to the treatment of phobias by systematic desensitization, in which the patient steadily learns to approach closer and closer to the phobic object or situation without ever experiencing a substantial level of fear.

A great deal of our experience and behaviour is determined by the treatment we receive from other people. Every pain patient knows how a row with family or friends will mysteriously awaken the pain experience in an acute form. It is as though an immature child within the otherwise mature adult were crying, 'You can't treat me like that – I've got an awful pain!' The social response of other people is perhaps the most powerful 'reward' of all, and hence it can either increase or decrease the experience of pain according to the individual's habitual social relations. Within the Washington rehabilitation department great attention is paid to training the staff and advising the patients' families on the best way of responding to the patients' general behaviour and complaints of pain. As described by Fordyce:

> Family members are instructed on how to 're-program' their responses regarding pain and well behaviour. This process requires systematic effort. It requires practice and repeated evaluation. For this reason it is important that when the patient enters a contingency management program for chronic pain key family members be available for frequent training sessions.
>
> Parallel to these approaches to the reduction of pain behaviour, effective treatment will require detailed attention to the well-behaviour repertoire of the patient. To leave to chance the replacement of pain behaviour by well behaviour is to court disaster.[16]

It will be apparent from the foregoing that in order to institute a therapeutic régime for patients suffering from chronic pain it is very necessary to keep ongoing records of all the factors relating to the patient's condition. These records are not kept simply for the benefit of the psychologists, physicians and nurses, but also for the patient himself, and he should be encouraged to study his daily chart, except in so far as drug dosages may be concerned. Indeed, the patient may be asked to monitor his own condition. The McGill-Melzack Pain Questionnaire, which is reproduced in Appendix 2, is generally accompanied by a Home Recording Card, which the patient completes on a quarter-daily basis. It enables both him and the pain clinic to monitor his progress, to modify his drug dosage and to adjust his activity levels and general management. Most pain clinics issue their patients with recording sheets of this nature.

Part of the purpose of such self-assessment relates to the process known as 'biofeedback', whereby one may do such apparently astonishing things as deliberately altering one's blood-pressure or changing the electrical rhythms of one's brain. Biofeedback depends upon immediate knowledge of results. For instance, Roberts and his associates found that subjects who could see small changes in their skin temperature on a visual display, could learn to modify the temperature by voluntary effort.[17] The mere fact of having immediate knowledge of progress enables people to take control of the course of that progress. Biofeedback as a means of achieving control over pain has been rather over-boosted by enthusiasts in the past, and indeed there has been strong encouragement from makers of commercial instruments,[18] but we can learn from the general field of this research.

The study of Fordyce et al., already referred to,[19] concerned a population of patients hospitalized for a variety of conditions of chronic pain, the majority of whom suffered from low-back pain. Precise records were kept of the patients' own assessment of their pain levels on a five-point scale, and there were objective records of the patients' activity levels, periods of rest, etc. The patients themselves, as well as the nursing and other staff, had a visible record of how their present experience related to their balance of activity and rest. Pain is very difficult to remember, and therefore immediate recording on a quantifiable scale is entirely necessary. In this régime the patients could see beyond all question that although they still suffered some pain, it was less than they previously suffered, and also that their activity had increased.

The training of the nursing staff included instruction in how they should act towards the patients. They were to praise the patients' efforts to be more active and to establish meaningful social relations with them so that their friendliness really was rewarding. Complaints about pain were to be listened to, but not be rewarded by increased social attention or special sympathy. *Complaining* was never rewarded by extra human warmth: the human warmth and concern had to manifest itself as an unconditional feature of the whole régime. Such withholding of sympathy in response to complaints of pain may seem harsh, but it is in the patients' best interest to break the vicious circle of pain-behaviour being rewarded by sympathetic indulgence, and hence more pain being generated.

Fordyce et al. report that this treatment régime resulted in a decrease in the level of pain reported, fewer demands for analgesics and greater daily activity, an improvement which was maintained after the discharge of the patients from hospital.

Improvement in Behaviour or Improvement in Experience?

We now come to a very controversial question in the treatment of chronic pain, the extent to which patients may be playing 'pain games', and the implications of this for therapy. If some patients are playing such 'games' they are presumed to be trapped by psychological mechanisms, the nature of which they are not wholly aware.

The concept of 'game playing' is entirely technical and must not be misunderstood in terms of amusement. It originated in the work of Eric Berne, and is set out in his influential book *Games People Play*.[20] A 'game' is an interpersonal transaction which serves ends ulterior to those which are immediately apparent, and only by reading the extensive literature which has grown up around this area of social psychology can one truly appreciate what is meant by 'games'. Definitions are seldom adequate, but Berne's own definition is as follows:

> A game is a ongoing series of complementary ulterior transactions progressing to a well-defined, predictable outcome. Descriptively it is a recurring set of transactions, often repetitious, superficially plausible, with a concealed motivation; or, more colloquially, a series of moves with a snare, or 'gimmick'. Games are clearly differentiated from procedures, rituals and pastimes by two chief characteristics: (1) their ulterior quality and (2) the payoff. Procedures may be successful, rituals effective and pastimes profitable, but all of them are by definition candid; they may involve contest, but not conflict, and the ending may be sensational, but it is not dramatic. Every game, on the other hand, is basically dishonest, and the outcome has a dramatic, as distinct from a merely exciting, quality.[21]

The theory of 'game playing' has been pursued in the study of therapy for chronic pain, notably by Richard Sternbach, a clinical psychologist. Greenhoot and Sternbach, in describing their therapeutic régime at the Pain Unit of the Veterans Administration Hospital, San Diego, write:

> The games represent behaviour which is useful to patients in manipulating others, using pain in the service of the interpersonal manipulation. The number of these 'games' and their variants is truly amazing. We have seen patients lie about the results of placebo anesthetic blocks in order to convince the surgeon that he should do what they know correctly from previous blocks should be done. We have seen patients use their pain as a retaliation against a spouse in a marriage that both parties wished dissolved long ago.[22]

This is strong stuff, and at once an objection may be raised to the presumption that 'patients lie about the results of placebo anesthetic blocks in order to convince the surgeon. . . .' A placebo anaesthetic block is an injection of a fluid which is, unknown to the patient, completely neutral, to see if he will respond in the same way as he did when a drug was injected. To assume that the patient is 'lying' is to make a huge assumption about the nature of placebo reactions; to assume, furthermore, that it is *motivated* lying is surely unwarranted. Elsewhere Sternbach admits that 'Not even the use of placebo analgesics or placebo blocks can serve to distinguish psychogenic from somatogenic pain since placebo responses can be obtained from a large proportion of patients with clearly identifiable lesions.'[23]

In Greenhoot and Sternbach's Pain Unit the patients attend daily group therapy sessions together with a psychologist, the nursing staff and, occasionally, the surgeon. According to these authors, 'The therapy consists of frank discussions of "pain games", of their use by patients in pain, and the ways in which they interfere with rehabilitation.'[24] They believe that the various 'games' that patients employ are most efficiently exposed by the other patients who used to employ such 'games' themselves. All this is somewhat reminiscent of psychodynamic group therapy, which takes place under the general psychoanalytic umbrella, and which may become a 'game' in itself. Once lay people have learnt a smattering of the jargon and some of the elementary Freudian concepts, they can play endlessly at attributing hidden motives to other people's actions, whatever they say or do. This activity has been well satirized by Stephen Potter in his 'gamesmanship' where the ultimate object is to come out 'one up'.

Although it is undisputed that some sufferers from chronic pain use their disability for the achievement of ulterior ends, it is legitimate to ask, 'And what ends are the therapists pursuing – the true end of effecting cure or alleviation of their patients' pain and invalid status, or the *appearance* of that end?'

Sternbach writes:

> Ultimately, most patients in our program make some improvement and are discharged. For those who do not receive surgery . . . the average length of stay is about 6 weeks; it is somewhat longer for those receiving surgery, counting convalescent and physical rehabilitation periods. At the end of their stay we have a little ceremony for public recognition of their improvement, and award them a certificate. . . . Occasionally a patient who plays the Confounder's game will not have benefited from his stay at all; he also will have earned a certificate of achievement. . . .[25]

The first of these certificates congratulates the patient on having 'learned to live well despite having pain and so is entitled to the greatest admiration and respect'. The second certificate can only be regarded as a document satirizing the 'failed' patient, a sort of dunce's cap. It certifies that he is a 'PERPETUAL PAIN PATIENT who has defeated the best efforts of our specialists and is to be congratulated on this achievement'. This document is highly significant; it denies the possibility that the failure of treatment is to be laid at the door of the specialists because of their incompetence, and places the blame squarely on the patient, implying that the fault is in his wilful determination to defeat his well-wishers.

This raises the important issue of whether the therapeutic régime outlined by Sternbach, when it appears to succeed, *really* alleviates the patients' pain, or whether it manipulates them by various psychological devices, including group pressure and the threat of the 'dunce's cap', into merely pretending that they have improved. Do some of the patients who publicly avow that they are better, privately admit that they have gained no benefit? Where the extent of real improvement is being masked by pseudo-improvement, then it is impossible to assess the effectiveness of the régime.

This point was raised by Martin Orne in discussion of the paper by Fordyce already referred to. Orne said:

I think some people get uncomfortable with the tendency to effect pain reports in which you really do not care whether or not it hurts. If someone is hurting and does not tell you about it, I believe he is still hurting, and maybe some of us would like to address this issue. I think everybody would agree that you must first remove the contingencies which pain effects. The second question then becomes, what are some of the specific things you can do to treat the experience of pain? I think that it is in this context that hypnosis may be useful.[26]

The effectiveness of hypnosis in the treatment of pain has already been discussed in Chapter 5. In fact, Fordyce does make some use of hypnosis, and in the discussion referred to above he stated:

We occasionally use hypnosis as part of our program. Not often, but the most direct application would be one in which we use hypnosis as a way of producing a deeper level of relaxation than the method I was describing a moment ago for pacers. It is also true that we are trying not only to reduce sick behavior, but also to increase well behavior. One might use hypnosis and other techniques as a means of increasing certain skills, such as social skills, or getting round certain interpersonal problems or personality conflicts, thereby facilitating well behavior.[27]

Sternbach also uses hypnosis, but apparently only for the purpose of enabling patients to get to sleep, and he reports, rather surprisingly, that in his programme, they 'keep no separate records which would permit its evaluation'.[28]

The régime outlined by Greenhoot and Sternbach has been criticized here because of the element of psychological pressure which may result in some patients falsifying their pain reports in the direction of publicly claiming to experience less pain than they really do, thus masking the extent of any real improvement with pseudo-improvement. In fairness, however, it must be pointed out that what these two therapists set out to do (and tell their patients so) is to change *behaviour*, not private experience. Greenhoot and Sternbach believe that the patients' behaviour is the only adequate measure of success or failure in pain relief. An ex-patient who does not function adequately although he has no pain they would regard as a 'bad result', whereas another who still experiences pain, but who 'lives well', they would judge a success in terms of rehabilitation. Whether one should be content with this limited aim, rather than attempting to do more to solve the problem of the subjective experience of pain, is another matter. No psychologist practising behaviour therapy would regard his treatment of a condition such as claustrophobia as very successful if he merely got the patient physically to enter closed places, whilst continuing to suffer agonies of terror every time he did so.

The Under-Active and the Over-Active Pain Patient

Most of the foregoing discussion envisages a type of patient who is under-active because it hurts him to move, and who does himself no good by spending too much time lying around when he would be better engaged in some physical activity. It seems a natural form of therapy for a patient whose chronic pain has originated with an injured back to rest a great deal. Nevertheless, as has been discussed, a state of pain may be maintained by rest becoming a 'reward' for pain, and controlled exercises may improve the condition and reduce the pain. The exercises developed by Williams and Worthingham[29] are advocated by Barbara DeLateur[30] in cases of low-back pain and spinal injury because they strengthen relevant muscle groups which help to keep the spine and pelvis in a proper position; a weakening of these muscles will lead to degenerative changes and throw too much strain on the intervertebral joints.

Although the régimes described by Fordyce and by Greenhoot and Sternbach assume that most chronic pain patients spend too much time resting, we must recognize the great differences between individual patients. Some patients are definitely over-active, and their pain problem relates partly to this over-activity. In the discussion quoted above, Fordyce referred to such over-active patients as 'pacers'; these are patients who tend to pace restlessly up and down the wards whilst others are relaxing. For such over-active people the assumption that rest is a 'reward' is doubtful. According to Fordyce, pacers have often conditions of high-back, neck and shoulder pain or tension headaches, and for them the usual procedure of rewarding work with rest can be reversed. They are only too keen to work, and they benefit from having to earn their work quota by fulfilling a required quota of rest. A form of therapy which is very appropriate for them is training in relaxation methods with biofeedback and hypnosis, and in such training they are taught to try to obtain certain specified levels of deep relaxation. Obviously, the number of hours spent lying down is of less importance than the amount of real relaxation that is achieved. If biofeedback is used, the relevant physiological measure to be monitored and communicated to the patient is the degree of muscle-tension, as measured by the EMG, which can be conveyed to the patient either as a visual display or as an auditory signal. Training involving giving patients knowledge of their alpha brain rhythm may also be helpful, for alpha rhythm is a good measure of general relaxation.[31] The alpha-training procedure involves subjects learning to put themselves into a 'meditational state' and has been tried, without a great deal of success, in treating chronic pain by Gannon and Sternbach.[32] This method was followed up by Melzack and Perry[33] who treated chronic pain patients with alpha training alone, with hypnotic training, and with a combination of both methods. The combination of the two methods was found to be the most effective in reducing pain, and Melzack is an eloquent advocate for the judicious combination of different methods of treatment by interdisciplinary co-operation in pain clinics.

The fact that under-activity is associated with the pain problems of some patients, and over-activity with the problems of others, is a salutary warning against treating all patients by the same methods simply because they all complain of the same type of pain originally acquired through the same type of injury.

In the earlier part of the 1970s régimes were set up in pain clinics and hospital wards based partly on the concept that chronic pain was subject to learning and unlearning according to the principles of operant conditioning. As we have seen, there is a suspicion that these therapeutic programmes merely inculcated a stoical attitude rather than actually reducing the levels of pain experienced. More recent research has shown that such a suspicion is not entirely justified: some patients do indeed greatly reduce their experience of pain, and continue to improve after they have finished the treatment. There remains, however, a group of patients who either do not benefit at all from the treatment, or who benefit during the period they are in the care of the clinic, but deteriorate after they have been discharged. The differences between these groups, the 'successes' and the 'failures', has now become a focus for research. When we know more about the personal factors associated with success or failure we will have advanced further along the road to solving the mystery of chronic pain.

Newman et al.[34] invited thirty-six ex-patients who had been treated for chronic low-back pain at their clinic to return ten months after discharge for assessment of progress. It was found that statistically significant gains had been achieved in the reduction of prescription analgesics, and on four measures of physical functioning. Most patients claimed that they were coping much better and were making far less use of medical resources for further pain treatment. This was indeed a vindication of the multidisciplinary approach to treatment which was in use at the clinic. However, a very strange finding emerged when the ex-patients were asked to compare their present pain experience with their level of pain on original admission. Their comparisons varied enormously, ranging between 80 per cent better and 80 per cent worse. Indeed, only a minority of this sample claimed that their pain level was now lower, even though the life-style of the group as a whole had improved, their physical activity had increased and their drug-taking had been greatly reduced. Here we are reminded of the distinction between 'pain' and 'suffering'; it is pertinent to suggest that these paradoxical results indicate that, as far as we can generalize about the group, their *suffering* had been substantially reduced whilst they still complained of *pain*. It has already been mentioned that after the neurosurgical operation of frontal lobotomy, patients say that they still feel the pain but it no longer distresses them.[35] This matter calls for a great deal of further research.

A later study at the same pain clinic[36] was directed to comparing those who maintained their progress after discharge with those who deteriorated. This was done by means of a postal questionnaire sent to 500 ex-patients, and as in all such studies, there was the drawback that only a minority of those polled returned their questionnaires. Considering those who responded, the pain clinic experience had been successful, rated about a year after discharge, for three-quarters of the patients. Of these a quarter reported that the gains had been wiped out with the passage of time. In order to investigate the factors associated with improvement or deterioration, twenty-five 'successes' were compared with twenty-five 'failures'. The complexity of all the relevant factors involved cannot be discussed here, but the general tendency was for those who had a greater *incentive* to recover to maintain their progress, whereas those who appeared to lack incentive deteriorated. If this seems curious – for what greater incentive may a person have than a nagging pain in the back? – the explanation would appear to be that the difference between striving hard and tamely accepting the status quo is not entirely a matter of deliberate choice; the 'rewards' of being a pain patient are seldom obvious to the patient himself.

What emerged from this study was a finding common to a number of other research studies (e.g. Block *et al.*)[37]: that those in receipt of disability payments because of their injury, deteriorated, *even though they had improved during the course of the therapy*. Another factor that emerged, and at first sight seems extraordinary, was that the status of being divorced or separated was positively and significantly associated with success. This finding is not easy to explain, but the authors of the study suggest that those who were free of marital ties (there were no single people in the study) would be more flexible in being able to adapt their life-style in accordance with the advice they had received, and to change their 'patterns of reinforcement'.

Related to the finding that incentive makes for continued improvement after discharge is the fact that the 'successes' improved considerably in mood during the course of therapy. At the beginning of the course they were equally or more depressed than those who were to become post-discharge failures, but they experienced a steady upswing of mood. The authors conclude:

> Perhaps the most striking differences among groups are reflected in the changes they report in life-style following treatment. Those who regress point to very little change in patterns of communication or reinforcement after they leave the program, suggesting that patterns which had previously supported pain behaviour continue to do so, contributing to regression to pre-treatment levels of function. The success group, on the other hand, shows considerable change.[38]

One gets the impression from this study that the stereotype of the 'failure' who regresses after an otherwise successful stay at the pain centre is someone who is unemployed but in receipt of a disability allowance, sitting quietly at home with a spouse, somewhat depressed and lacking the incentive or initiative to make much change in life – a sad but cosy condition which is supported by the family. Freud's concept of dammed-up libido being transmuted to pain does not seem inappropriate here. The 'success' who can benefit from the therapeutic programme and make continued gains, seems to be someone who may have to respond to the incentive of economic pressure by getting a job, and is adventurous even to the extent of breaking matrimonial ties. Obviously these are merely clues which call for further investigation.

Programmes for therapy need not necessarily involve in-patient treatment or take up much time of various specialists, even when they are interdisciplinary. A recent study has been published by a physiotherapist and an occupational therapist who have backgrounds in psychology and psychiatry. They run a clinic where there is the occasional back-up help from specialists in neurosurgery, anaesthesiology, biofeedback, hypnosis and psychotherapy, as required.[39] They organized 'pain control classes' which ran for units of nine weeks, catering for groups of between twelve and fourteen patients. Seventy-five patients have now completed these classes, and the results indicate a drop in *pain perception*, as well as in depression of mood and analgesic intake. Employment figures increased from 20 per cent to 48 per cent after completion of the programme. Nevertheless, sixteen of the seventy-five patients were regarded as 'failures', and the study throws further light on the factors which make for success or failure, prominent among them being the deleterious effect of being in receipt of compensation for injury or having litigation pending. This sounds as though such patients were malingering, but all the evidence points away from such a simplistic conclusion. There is good evidence for believing that a quite genuine state of pain is maintained by actual or potential economic reward.

The question of individual differences in pain and suffering is a very important one, and applies equally to acute, transient pains and to chronic pain. These individual differences are as yet imperfectly understood, and, as we have stressed earlier, further progress in the treatment of pain states necessitates close study of such differences.

In discussing chronic pain, we have concentrated on the condition of chronic low-back pain because it is by far the most common condition which comes to the attention of the therapeutic services. According to Devlin,[40] every year one in twenty-five people in Britain goes to the doctor about back pain, and it costs the country £300,000,000 a year in medical care, sickness benefit and lost production. What goes for low-back pain also goes for other conditions of chronic pain in general, with regard to the circumstances which exacerbate them and the forms of therapy that are available. There is, however, one condition which (partly because of its fearsome reputation, the name itself striking some people with quite irrational terror) deserves to be considered separately: that of painful cancer.

Cancer

This is a book about the nature and treatment of pain, and not about physical and psychological illnesses; consequently, it would be quite inappropriate to attempt to discuss the nature and treatment of cancer in any detail. The topic must be mentioned, however, because people have quite exaggerated ideas about the association of pain with cancer, and some hypochondriacal individuals live in fear that they will end their days racked with chronic pain, while doctors mutter to their sorrowing relatives, 'Hush - it's c*****!' It seems advisable, therefore, to say a few words about cancer and the extent to which it may give rise to chronic pain.

The statistics are undeniable; about 20 per cent of us will die of cancer,[41] and if this seems a shocking statistic, let us remember that 100 per cent of us will die of *something*, and among the 80 per cent of us who will die of other causes, some will have conditions rather more uncomfortable, painful and generally distressing than those experienced by the cancer sufferers. In saying that one in five of us 'will' die of cancer we are being deliberately pessimistic: this is the present prospect, given current social conditions and extent of medical knowledge. If these improve, then the rate of death from cancer will decline, and more of us will have to die from other causes, including sheer senility. But the reason why cancer has as high a death rate as it stands at present, is partly due to psychological causes - that people have a totally irrational fear of the disease. This fear prevents people from seeking help *early*, before the disease has made much headway and the chance of complete cure is greater. According to Ian Burn, Consultant Surgeon at Charing Cross Hospital, London:

Fear is frequently the cause for delay. The woman who delays seeking advice for a lump in the breast usually does so because she is so frightened that it may be cancer that she cannot bring herself to face the diagnosis. Usually at some stage, and often after a delay of months, she is able to overcome her fear to a point that medical advice is sought, but by then it may be too late even to attempt a curative procedure. The fear is usually of the cancer and the apparent inevitability of death rather than the mastectomy which might be advised if the diagnosis is made. In general, we have failed to communicate widely enough that the cancerous diseases can be cured if treated early and . . . this is paralleled by the fact that even among the caring professions there remains widespread ignorance of the results of treatment.[42]

If psychological attitudes of fear and misunderstanding contribute to the death rate from cancer, they undoubtedly also contribute to the amount of pain which is associated with the disease, as will be demonstrated later.

Regarding the association of cancer with pain, we may quote the authority of an eminent oncologist, R. B. Scott: 'It is difficult to explode the myth that cancer is inevitably painful.'[43] Indeed, it is a pity that cancer is *not* inevitably a painful disease, for then people would seek to do something about it in its early stages and cure would be easier. Whether or not it is painful in its later stages depends very much on the site and the type of the cancerous condition. Pain may be caused by a tumour pressing upon neighbouring nerves, or by the infiltration of cancer cells from the tumour into neighbouring tissue, affecting the nerve fibres. Where the affected organ is one such as the mouth, which is constantly mobile, the condition is naturally painful. It will be remembered that Sigmund Freud suffered from cancer of the mouth for the last sixteen years of his life, but he lived until the age of eighty-three and, although he endured many operations, the 'sore mouth' of which he complained did not inhibit him from talking and lecturing.

One of the well-known features of cancer is that the primary tumour of cancerous cells can have small groups of these cells carried away in the bloodstream or lymph vessels to lodge elsewhere in the body and continue growing. Such colonies are known as 'metastases', and it is these secondary deposits that are more likely to cause pain. A somewhat infrequent occurrence is for a metastasis to cause a breakdown of a spinal vertebra, and hence the usual problems of back-ache arise acutely. A vaguely painful state may characterize the really advanced condition of 'cachexia' when the disease has gone so far that the patient is anaemic, wasted and apathetic, slowly dying from all the multifarious effects. How much of this pain is inevitable, and how much the general psychological result of a long-endured stress which is preventable, is a matter for discussion.

In advanced cases of cancer, as pointed out by Moricca,[44] the patient's health is being attacked by three different factors: the disease, the pain caused by the disease and the drugs which are used to combat the pain. The patient who has come to accept that his life expectancy is severely limited by the disease, must take some very positive decisions about his way of life. He may decide that the problem is not so much one of adding extra days to his life, as enriching the quality of his life for the remainder of his days. Certainly if pain is present, that is the major problem, but he should understand that pain can be minimized by methods other than by narcotics. A proper programme of pain-control, according to the principles already discussed in this book, must be worked out. An enriched life is not only valuable in itself, but it will lead to a lesser experience of pain.

One bogy associated with cancer is the prospect of becoming addicted to narcotic drugs prescribed for the relief of pain, so that even if the condition is controlled or cured, and the patient has a long expectancy of life, he will become a confirmed drug addict. This fear is less justified nowadays because we know more about the treatment of pain by surgical, pharmacological and psychological means. Dosing with narcotics has become partly replaced by the use of psychotropic drugs, that is, drugs which do not have a directly narcotizing or analgesic effect, but which act upon the psychological mood state. Generally they are given in various combinations, and therapeutic skill consists in finely adjusting the dosages to suit the individual patient. If we knew more about the essential psychological factors which make for different drug-responses in people of different personality, this matter could be even more skilfully controlled. The psychotropic drugs alter our perception, and hence the manner in which we process sensory stimuli, and whether we experience them as painful or not. Kocher has referred to this phenomenon as 'the de-personalization of pain';[45] it is similar to that already discussed regarding the attenuation of acute pain by hypnosis, or the treatment of chronic pain by frontal leucotomy. The extent to which psychotropic drugs may have a peripheral action and actually interfere with the synthesis and elimination of pain-producing chemical substances, is not definitely established. It is generally held, however, that such psychotropic drugs as the phenothiazines potentiate the action of narcotics.

According to Orne,[46] patients with severe pain can tolerate very high dosages of phenothiazines and function quite well with them. If the cancer condition is ameliorated by therapy, thus reducing the severity of the pain, the patient will then become very drowsy unless the phenothiazine dosage is immediately reduced.

Orne recommends a multi-disciplinary approach to the treatment of cancer patients, using hypnosis in addition to pharmacological agents for the relief of pain. A programme of teaching the patient techniques of self-hypnosis will enable him to cut down on the dosage of drugs, and generally raise his morale. Whatever the prognosis of the cancer condition, there is a definite gain to be made in the reduction of pain, the increase in the patient's enjoyment of food, social interaction, reading and other recreations, and in encouraging him to be as active as he can in looking after himself.

Paradoxically, in the article under discussion, Orne argues that although hypnosis is appropriate for conditions of pain which are clearly organic in origin, such as those which may arise from cancer, it is less appropriate and may indeed be contra-indicated when the pain is functional. Orne writes as follows:

> To the extent that functional pain serves an important need, it is necessary for the patient to develop alternative mechanisms or alternative symptoms. Management by psychological methods other than hypnosis is generally desirable when it is clear that the pain is used in the service of significant interpersonal needs.[47]

This raises the controversial distinction between organic and functional pain which is not wholly accepted in this book. Rather we would say that a *condition* may be largely organic or largely functional, but that the *pain* arising from that condition is always a functional phenomenon. Cancer is certainly an organic condition, but any one of us who suffers chronic pain from that condition will use it, to some extent, 'in the service of significant interpersonal needs', and we should not be ashamed to admit the fact. When we shout at the children, snap at the wife and are rude to our friends, excusing ourselves because of this nasty pain, we are doing just that. If we have to endure this horrid ache, we might as well use it! No one becomes a saint simply because he has cancer. Orne's argument is simply a legacy from the old Freudian era, in which it was held that the patient 'needed' his symptoms, even if they included an atrocious pain.

It should be pointed out that neither Orne, nor any other reputable psychiatrist, psychoanalytic or otherwise, holds that the cancer patient should be left in his pain because he 'needs' it. At the extreme of the psychoanalytic school was Wilhelm Reich, who in his book *The Cancer Biopathy*[48] claimed that the disease of cancer, and the pains it generated, were simply due to 'chronic sexual starvation'. Although few informed people will take Reich very seriously today, it must be pointed out that there is a huge variety of eccentric theories concerning the origins of cancer, and an equally wide variety of quack remedies for its cure, ranging from grape-juice to mistletoe.[49] One possible reason for the belief in the efficacy of the many weird remedies for cancer prescribed by unorthodox practitioners is the pain syndrome in the disease. Cancer sufferers who experience pain (and Twycross[50] points out that about 50 per cent of cancer patients do suffer from some degree of pain) come to identify their disease with the pain, and if they take some strange preparation in the confident belief that it may cure their cancer, their pain will indeed be relieved, sometimes to a dramatic extent, as long as their belief lasts.

UNNECESSARY PAIN

It has been demonstrated that just as pain can be relieved by the psychological mechanism of a placebo, so it can be disastrously increased by the psychological mechanisms of anxiety, depression and despair. Where pain occurs in cancer much of it is *unnecessary*, in the sense that it is the product of the attitude to the disease held by the patient, his family and his doctor. How much the success or failure of cancer therapy depends upon the attitude of the doctor, which gets conveyed to the patient, was shown by experiments on the 'Berkley-Smythe effect'.[51]

Berkley-Smythe was the pseudonym adopted by an enthusiastic thoracic surgeon in a cancer research project at McMaster University of Toronto, who utilized a vaccine for patients with lung cancer. Because of the remarkable degree of success which was associated with his breezily cheerful attitude towards treatment of the disease, the study was greatly expanded, but now carried out by different staff physicians. Unfortunately, some of them could not live up to the matter-of-fact cheerfulness of the required persona of 'Berkley-Smythe' and let their own depressed attitudes to the dread disease show through, and their patients did not do so well.

To what degree then is the pain associated with some cancers unnecessary? Research would indicate that a great deal of it is unnecessary. The great need is to de-mystify cancer, to undermine the awful image it has acquired in modern society, which is reminiscent of the irrational attitudes expressed towards leprosy in medieval times. There are indeed signs that this welcome development is taking place, and that enlightenment is coming to the people who count most, the patients and their families. Barbara Cox[52] has described the various self-help groups which are springing up, and she makes the important point that for too long cancer patients, whether suffering from serious or comparatively trivial conditions, have been the *passive* recipients of various therapies. Such passivity at the hands of the 'experts' can lead to a condition of clinical depression designated by Seligman[53] as 'learned helplessness', and such depression leads to the experience of severe chronic pain.

All that has been said about pain in this book applies to cancer as to any other condition which may generate pain. Cancer pains are not in a class of their own. This section has been written with the express purpose of showing that if pain is generated by cancer it is no different from the pain of toothache, stomach-ache or a 'slipped disc'.

REFERENCES

1 J. J. Bonica, 'Introduction', in J. J. Bonica and D. Albe-Fessard (eds), *Advances in Pain Research and Therapy*, op. cit.

2 See S. Freud, 'The economic problem of masochism', in L. and V. Woolf (eds), *Collected Papers*, Vol. II, London: Hogarth Press, 1942.

3 J. Breuer and S. Freud, 'Studies on hysteria' in J. Strachey (ed.), *Complete Works of Sigmund Freud*, op. cit.

4 H. Merskey and F. G. Spear, *Pain: Psychological and Psychiatric Aspects*, op. cit.

5 See the following: E. Rudinger, *Avoiding Back Trouble*, London: Consumers' Association, 1975; P. Gillan and R. Gillan, *Sex Therapy Today*, London: Open Books, 1976; S. Fisher, *Understanding the Female Orgasm*, Harmondsworth: Penguin Books, 1973.

6 B. F. Skinner, *Science and Human Behavior*, op. cit.

7 See N. E. Miller, 'Learning of visceral and glandular responses', *Science*, 1969, 163, pp. 434–45.

8 N. E. Miller and A. Banuazizi, 'Instrumental learning by curarized rats of a specific visceral response', *Journal of Comparative Physiological Psychology*, 1968, 65, pp. 1–7.

9 W. E. Fordyce, 'Pain viewed as learned behaviour', in J. J. Bonica (ed.), *Advances in Neurology*, op. cit., p. 418.

10 Ibid., p. 419.

11 For a discussion of the innate basis of fears which may generate phobias, see S. Rachman, *The Meanings of Fear*, Harmondsworth: Penguin Books, 1974, Chap. 5.

12 See H. J. Eysenck, 'The conditioning model of neurosis', *Brain and Behavior Sciences*, 1979, 2, pp. 155–99.

13 F. J. Evans, 'The placebo response in pain reduction', in J. J. Bonica (ed.), *Advances in Neurology*, op. cit., p. 296.

14 See W. E. Fordyce, R. S. Fowler Jr., J. F. Lehman, B. J. DeLateur, P. L. Sand and R. B. Trieschman, 'Operant conditioning in the treatment of chronic pain', *Archives of Physical Medicine and Rehabilitation*, 1973, 54, pp. 399–408.

15 See B. S. Glick and R. Margolis, 'A study of the influence of experimental design on clinical outcome in drug research', *American Journal of Psychiatry*, 1962, 118, pp. 1087–96.

16 W. E. Fordyce, 'Treating chronic pain by contingency management', in J. J. Bonica (ed.), *Advances in Neurology*, op. cit., p. 588.

17 A. H. Roberts, J. Shuler, J. G. Bacon, R. L. Zimmerman and R. Patterson, 'Individual differences and autonomic control: Absorption, hypnotic susceptibility and the unilateral control of skin temperature', *Journal of Abnormal Psychology*, 1975, 84, pp. 272–9.

18 See R. Melzack, 'The promise of biofeedback: Don't hold the party yet,' *Psychology Today*, 1975, 9, p. 18.

19 W. E. Fordyce *et al.*, 'Operant conditioning in the treatment of chronic pain', op. cit.

20 E. Berne, *Games People Play: The Psychology of Human Relationships*, London: André Deutsch, 1966.

21 Ibid., p. 48.

22 J. H. Greenhoot and R. A. Sternbach, 'Conjoint treatment of chronic pain', in J. J. Bonica (ed.), *Advances in Neurology*, op. cit. pp. 598–9.

23 R. A. Sternbach, 'Psychological factors in pain', in J. J. Bonica and D. Albe-Fessard (eds), *Advances in Pain Research and Therapy*, op. cit., p. 297.

24 J. H. Greenhoot and R. A. Sternbach, 'Conjoint treatment in chronic pain', op. cit., p. 599.

25 R. A. Sternbach, *Pain Patients: Traits and Treatments*, op. cit., p. 106.

26 M. T. Orne, 'Floor discussion of operant conditioning', in J. J. Bonica (ed.), *Advances in Neurology*, op. cit., p. 592.

27 W. E. Fordyce, ibid., pp. 591-2.

28 R. A. Sternbach, *Pain Patients: Traits and Treatments*, op. cit., p. 116.

29 M. Williams and C. Worthingham, *Therapeutic Exercises*, Philadelphia: W. B. Saunders & Co., 1957.

30 B. J. DeLateur, 'The role of physical medicine in problems of pain', in J. J. Bonica (ed.), *Advances in Neurology*, op. cit.

31 See J. Kamiya, 'Operant control of the E.E.G. alpha rhythm and some of its reported effects on consciousness', in C. T. Tart (ed.), *Altered States of Consciousness*, New York: Wiley, 1969.

32 L. Gannon and R. A. Sternbach, 'Alpha enhancement as a treatment for pain: A case study', *Journal of Behavior Therapy and Experimental Psychiatry*, 1971, 2, pp. 209-13.

33 R. Melzack and C. Perry, 'Self regulation of pain: the use of alpha feedback and hypnotic training for the control of chronic pain', *Experimental Neurology*, 1975, 46, pp. 452-69.

34 R. I. Newman, J. L. Seres, L. P. Yospe and B. Garlington, 'Multidisciplinary treatment of chronic pain: long-term follow-up of low-back patients', *Pain*, 1974, 4, pp. 283-92.

35 See A. Petrie, *Personality and the Frontal Lobes*, op. cit.

36 See J. R. Painter, J. L. Seres and R. I. Newman, 'Assessing the benefits of the pain center: why some patients regress', *Pain*, 1980, 8, pp. 101-13.

37 A. R. Block, E. Kremer and M. Gaylor, 'Behavioural treatment of chronic pain: variables affecting treatment efficacy', *Pain*, 1980, 8, pp. 367-75.

38 J. R. Painter, J. L. Seres and R. I. Newman, 'Assessing the benefits of the pain center: why some patients regress', op. cit., p. 111.

39 See E. Herman and S. Baptiste, 'Pain control: mastery through group experience', *Pain*, 1981, 10, pp. 79-86.

40 D. Devlin, *You and Your Back*, London: Pan Books, 1977.

41 See R. B. Scott, *Cancer: The Facts*, London: Oxford University Press, 1979.

42 I. Burn, 'Cancer education and treatment – the public', in R. W. Raven, *Outlook on Cancer*, London: Plenum Press, 1977, p. 128.

43 R. B. Scott, op. cit., p. 36.

44 G. Moricca, 'Pituitary neuroadenolysis in the treatment of intractible pain from cancer', in S. Lipton (ed.), *Persistent Pain: Modern Methods of Treatment*, London: Academic Press, 1977.

45 R. Kocher, 'Use of psychotropic drugs in the treatment of chronic severe pain', in J. J. Bonica and D. Albe-Fessard (eds), *Advances in Pain Research and Therapy*, op. cit.

46 M. T. Orne, 'Pain suppression by hypnosis and related phenomena', in J. J. Bonica (ed.), *Advances in Neurology*, op. cit.

47 Ibid., p. 571.

48 W. Reich, *The Cancer Biopathy* (1948), London: Vision Press, 1971.

49 For a compendium of quack remedies for cancer see M. Finkel, *Fresh Hope in Cancer*, Bradford: Holdsworthy Press, 1978.

50 R. G. Twycross, 'Relief of pain,' in C. M. Saunders (ed.), *The Management of Terminal Disease*, London: Edward Arnold, 1978, p. 66.

51 See P. J. Rosch, 'Cancer: a disease of adaptation?', in J. Taché, H. Seyle and S. B. Day (eds), *Cancer, Stress and Death*, New York.; Plenum Medical Book Co., 1979.

52 B. Cox, 'The cancer patient as educator and counsellor', ibid.

53 M. E. P. Seligman, 'Depression and learned helplessness', in R. J. Friedman and M. M. Katz (eds), *The Psychology of Depression: Contemporary Theory and Research*, Washington, D.C.: Winston-Wiley, 1975.

8

WOMEN'S PAINS

This chapter concerns a class of pain which has the unusual distinction of being associated with perfectly normal physiological functions. Some people regard this class of pain as unnatural, maintaining that the body has developed on the plan that its normal functioning, involving such operations as digestion, breathing, defaecation and muscular movement, does not cause pain unless there is some disease process at work. However, healthy women may, and frequently do, experience pain in association with menstruation, ovulation and childbirth. There are considerable individual differences between women as to the extent such pains are experienced, and a great deal of controversy exists as to the origins of women's pains, and the measures that should be taken to overcome them.

The feminist movement, which has taken quite different forms in different historical epochs, has naturally been concerned about women's pains and has advocated different remedial approaches. In the nineteenth century, for instance, feminists strongly advocated pharmacological remedies for obstetric pain, but the modern feminist movement is advocating a more psychological approach. Feminist agitation has secured various useful reforms in the health care of women; Florence Nightingale and her associates forced the medical profession to institute proper education in obstetric nursing and better training for midwives, and now the feminist movement is challenging what they see as an unnecessary hegemony of doctors in gynaecology and obstetrics. The degree to which feminist ideology and its converse affects the experience of pain and the relevant welfare of women will be discussed in this chapter, which seeks to explore the relevant theoretical issues and to provide the reader with a wide bibliography. In addition, we shall offer some practical suggestions, from a psychological point of view, as to how women can best meet the problems of pain which they may encounter by reason of their sex.

Dysmenorrhoea

The incidence of painful periods in women who have no particular gynaecological abnormality has been variously estimated by different researchers. Gregory[1] published estimates of between 1 per cent and 34 per cent; Coppen and Kessel[2] in a study involving nearly 500 menstruating women, found the incidence of severe pain to be 12 per cent, and moderate pain 46 per cent. They therefore concluded that the pain could not be considered as 'abnormal'. As to the cause and significance of dysmenorrhoea, some writers have let their theoretical orientations guide their speculations rather more than any considerations of controlled research. Wittowker and Wilson[3] suggested that the experience of pain in menstruation was associated with a difficulty in the acceptance of the feminine role. One might turn this speculation round and suggest an alternative view – that girls unlucky enough to have physical constitutions predisposing them to experience much menstrual pain on reaching puberty, would be more likely to resent their femininity as a direct result of this unfortunate experience.

According to Anne Broadhurst,[4] there is manifest throughout the literature a conflict of opinion between psychiatrists and gynaecologists, the former tending to the opinion that dysmenorrhoea is a sign of a neurotic personality, the latter maintaining that the psychogenic component is unimportant. Broadhurst is concerned mainly with British gynaecologists; by contrast, Paula Weideger,[5] an American feminist writer, maintains that in the USA there are many gynaecologists who take a superficial, psychodynamic view of female pains and are only too ready to cover up their own diagnostic incompetence by attributing women's pains to neurotic hang-ups. According to Ruzek, another American feminist:

> Recent medical texts' portrayal of dysmenorrhoea is illustrative both of physicians' attitudes towards women's reproductive disorders and textbook writers' unrealistic expectations of how clinicians practice in reality. Rather than focus on the organic bases of dysmenorrhoea, textbook authors suggest that primary management of dysmenorrhoea should be 'directed at the underlying psychodynamics'.[6]

In the Coppen and Kessel study the 500 women were taken from the lists of ten general practitioners and sent a questionnaire on menstrual symptoms, together with the Maudsley Personality Inventory (MPI). A high response rate of 93 per cent was obtained, and it was found that dysmenorrhoea was not related to neuroticism in terms of the MPI, but that neuroticism was significantly related to symptoms of the pre-menstrual syndrome such as irritability, depression and headache. We have observed in this book how the experience of any sort of pain is rather more severe in people who are higher on neuroticism, so this study tends to emphasize the point that menstrual pain is not itself a psychogenic symptom indicative of neuroticism. This study was replicated with students in Spain by Théano,[7] who found very similar results.

There is some evidence that girls tend to grow out of their painful periods. Thus Moos,[8] studying 839 wives of graduate students, found that the younger women complained of more pain at the onset of the period, whereas the older women were more concerned with the pre-menstrual symptoms.

Although dysmenorrhoea is seldom a manifestation of psychological disorder, in some cases it can be effectively treated by psychological means. The nature of the pain itself is complex and not entirely understood; there are many types of dysmenorrhoea, but it is commonly a pain of *ischemia*, the result of the womb contracting fiercely as in a cramp in other muscles. According to Dalton,[9] there are two main syndromes of dysmenorrhoeic pain, the *cramping* which starts on the first day of the flow and comes and goes in waves, and the *congestive* which is a dull, aching pain. It is likely that the former will be the more amenable to conditioning therapy. To the extent that it may be a conditioned pain, the pre-menstrual symptoms act as prodromal stimuli which precipitate the expected response, and as with other pains that have a learned component, it can be treated by psychological means as well as by drugs and hormonal preparations. Dorcus and Kirkner[10] make the important point that the treatment of pain by hypnosis is far more effective when the pain condition is episodic rather than continuous. They worked with two groups of patients, five males suffering from pain associated with spinal injuries, and five females suffering from dysmenorrhoea. The spinal cases were given, on average, sixteen sessions of therapeutic hypnosis each, and the dysmenorrhoea patients had from one to five hypnotic sessions each. While both groups benefited from the therapy to some degree, the authors reported that the dysmenorrhoeic group were 'relatively free from pain on discontinuance of therapy and have remained relatively free from pain for at least two years'.

This study illustrates the point that dysmenorrhoea often has a large component of learned pain, and should therefore be expected to yield to the conditioning therapies which have been developed by the behaviour therapists. While there are sporadic reports of such treatment (e.g. Mullen)[11] a search of the vast literature on behaviour therapy and the treatment of pain reveals that this condition, which is so very common in half the population, is seldom mentioned at all. We may contrast this with the much greater frequency of mention in the literature of female *dyspareunia* (painful sexual intercourse), a condition which naturally upsets the male partner and attracts considerable attention. This astonishing finding perhaps relates to the tradition of male dominance in the medical profession and, to some degree, in clinical psychology. Thus the post-pubertal girl who complains of painful periods is not likely to have her condition treated very seriously, merely being encouraged to 'grin and bear it'. Where organic conditions have definitely been ruled out, such lack of over-concern is not entirely to be deplored, for as already discussed in relation to conditions of chronic pain, if the onset of pain is always 'rewarded' by too much sympathy and coddling, then subsequent episodes may become more and more severe, for reasons given by Fordyce and his colleagues.[12] Nevertheless, such abstention from over-concern does not in any way justify the current lack of research into dysmenorrhoea, or the failure to use and develop the remedial psychological techniques for its control which have already been shown to be effective.

The post-pubertal girl must come to terms with the fact that she will continue to have a potentially painful condition for the rest of her fertile life, but this does not imply a passive acceptance of pain. Weideger, who discussed the nature of the taboos surrounding menstruation in various cultures, has expressed the position thus:

> Women don't have to accept pain, discomfort and the many side effects of hormonal change. Certainly minor problems with menstruation and menopause can be endured, but when they are no longer exacerbated by negative cultural stereotypes, they may be less painful. . . . Painless menstruation or symptom-free menopause are sound goals for medical research, but they ought not to be moral ideals. Perfection of the female spirit will not cure all ills, whether perfection is defined by a gynecologist or a woman. Any woman who is suffering from menstrual or menopausal problems has the right to relief and cure of these discomforts, and such remedies must be rigorously sought after. A woman is not born to suffer (or overcome suffering through moral perfection) any more than she is born unclean. While there is plenty of evidence that women have remarkable capacities to endure pain, there is no evidence that we are born masochists or saints. Female masochism appears to be one more male fantasy rationalizing male inattention to women's needs, and female 'bravery' appears to be the women's counterpart to the concept of masochism.[13]

Weidiger is a committed feminist and her protest against the cavalier attitude to menstrual pain adopted by some members of the medical profession is voiced by other writers from the feminist movement. The purpose of the present discussion is to make the point that if an area of human behaviour and experience is associated with shame, anxiety, worry and negative expectancy, even mild stress which might otherwise be quite exciting and pleasurable, will generate pain. The girl's experience of coming to terms with the potentially painful experience of menstruation, will be a learning experience in coming to terms with other experiences which may cause pain.

Finally, mention must be made of *mittelschmerz*, the pain which may develop about the fourteenth day of the menstrual cycle, and is assumed to be due to ovulation. Very little is known about the incidence of this sort of pain, and many women have never heard of it as a recognizable phenomenon. It may be that it is commoner than is supposed, but because it is not well known as a definite symptom, it is seldom reported by women who suffer from it. Were it reported more often and women expected their doctors to try to do something about it, then some useful research into the condition might be initiated.

The Pain of Childbirth

If the pain experienced in menstruation is to some degree dependent on expectations engendered by social attitudes, attitudinal factors apply equally to the pain of childbirth. Here we are on controversial ground, and must acknowledge that the politics of 'sexism' and 'radical feminism' unquestionably affect the different slants which are put upon the available evidence. On the one hand we have the argument that obstetric pain and distress are largely culturally determined, and evidence is advanced relating to cultures where childbirth is regarded in a manner very different from our own. On the other hand, there is the more traditional view that human anatomy having evolved as it has, considerable pain may naturally be expected in childbirth and there is nothing much that can be done about it.

Kroeber[14] presents evidence from various anthropological studies concerning the practice of the *couvade* in which the parturient mothers are assumed to experience very little pain in childbirth, and where they are expected to continue with their normal work until actually confined, and to return to work shortly after delivery. The bizarre feature of the *couvade* is that the husband takes on the role of enacting great pain, and may even stay in bed with the baby after the mother has returned to work. This is not, as it sometimes supposed, a rare aberration among a group of very primitive peoples who may even differ physically from modern Europeans, but a custom found in many different parts of the world. It was practised in Corsica in the first century AD, and also in Spain and Cyprus. It is reported to have occurred in the twentieth century in Holland and in the Baltic States, in the Congo, among the Japanese Ainu, and in quite unrelated races all over the world. Essentially, therefore, it is a social custom and it demonstrates the immense variability of adaptation to childbirth that is determined by prior social expectation. Either one can regard it as yet another flagrant imposition on long-suffering womanhood by sexist men, or as a clever feminist ploy to make men accept their role of responsible paternity, and to experience some of the pain of labour. As to whether men really do experience pain in the *couvade*, there is considerable evidence that expectant fathers around the time of childbirth (in societies where the *couvade* is not practised) sometimes experience strange psychosomatic pains. There is no doubt about the reality of this strange phenomenon, which has been well documented.[15] It has found its place in British folklore to the extent that a man's true paternity of his putative offspring may be doubted if he does not experience pain during his wife's confinement.

But if fathers really do experience pain during the *couvade*, as most authorities aver, do the mothers experience less pain than is normal in our modern culture? Various authorities interpret the evidence differently: Melzack, for instance, states that 'the women show virtually no distress during childbirth'. We might feel more confident about this if we could actually ask the women rather than merely observe the custom.

Some writers have suggested that childbirth in less developed societies is comparatively painless, and that it is only among civilized women that painful labour occurs. The wide survey of childbirth in many different cultures given by Chertok[16] does not support this idea. Freedman and Ferguson[17] bring forward evidence to show that while childbirth practices vary enormously among different peoples, their 'primitiveness' is not associated with easier labour. Our own Christian-Judaic culture not only assumes that childbirth will be extremely painful, but that such pain is ordained as a punishment for the daughters of Eve, as justified in the text of Genesis 3: 16, quoted earlier.

THE FEMINIST PROTEST

Before we discuss the methods which have been developed for the psychological control of obstetric pain and the general management of childbirth, it will be as well to consider the attitudes expressed by the feminist movement to the whole process.

The models of obstetric care have been set out by one American feminist writer, Ruzek,[18] who describes four models of health care operating in relation to obstetrics and gynaecology: (i) the traditional-authoritarian; (ii) the traditional-egalitarian; (iii) the traditional-feminist, and (iv) the radical-feminist. In so far as these four models exist in practice, or at least may come into being, they are worth considering as a basis for discussing relevant feminist attitudes.

(i) The *traditional-authoritarian* model operates in many clinics and hospitals, particularly where less educated women receive care. Such clinics are dominated by physicians who believe that obstetric patients should show a willingness to relinquish control to the doctor and refrain from seeking too many explanations. In such a setting women are expected to be passive and not to function as competent adults. Such a setting may in fact suit some women, who expect doctors to behave in this way, and feel safe in their hands, but as Arms[19] points out, many childbearing women have to go along with such procedures because they have little choice. In régimes of this kind heavy dosages of analgesic drugs are likely to be given to parturient women routinely, whether they are necessary or not.

(ii) In the *traditional-egalitarian* setting physicians are more ready to answer questions and give the mothers reasons why they are expected to follow the directions they are given. Here the physicians appreciate the value of intelligent co-operation on the part of their patients, while reserving to themselves the final arbitration as to what is to be done. Such a régime is more likely to be observed in hospital or home deliveries where women are middle class.

(iii) In *traditionalist-feminist* settings the role of female ancillary staff such as nurses and midwives is likely to be enhanced, and that of the physician minimized. This 'ideal' setting of an all-female community caring for a parturient woman has traditional roots in those cultures which seek to exclude men from the birth process, and it is interesting that there is a move to introduce it to our own. Female doctors fit into such settings, but there is nevertheless a feeling that the traditions of the medical profession are so strong that all medical doctors incline to a masculine authoritarianism.

Even in the West, at some historical times men have been forbidden to assist in accouchement. Later, in the years 1900–1930, as documented by Barker-Benfield,[20] American physicians made a strong bid entirely to take over the role of midwives and oust the latter from their livelihood. As late as 1958 it is stated in a nursing textbook that in America:

> The training of nursing in midwifery has been prevented by the attitude of the medical profession, who have held the ideal that every woman should be aided in delivery by a physician. In actual fact, thousands of women live where no doctor is available;

thousands more are delivered accidentally by nurses trained only in obstetrical nursing; other thousands employ incompetent midwives.[21]

In Britain, and in most other European countries, the position has been different, the physicians seeking to train and control midwives as an ancillary profession.

It is paradoxical that the modern feminist movement, which advocates freedom of expression for women and the end of the sex taboos which were formerly used to keep women in a spiritual purdah, should now be advocating as one of the reasons for creating an all-female environment for the rite of childbirth that 'an all-female staff (including physicians) is critical for creating an atmosphere where questions can be asked without embarrassment'.[22] So much for the alleged demise of Victorian prudery!

One good aspect of this traditionalist-feminist setting for the welfare of the mother is that women are expected to assume more responsibility for their own health care. This is an entirely laudable end, for the whole history of medicine shows that general increases in health have resulted from social developments in public health rather than from progress in 'disease medicine'. As far as pain in childbirth is concerned, it seems likely that the woman who is managing her own affairs rather than 'putting herself in the hands of a doctor', and who has had this expectation during pregnancy, will be better able to undergo labour with minimal pain.

The most obvious disadvantage of the setting just described is the exclusion of the father of the child. Without returning to the *couvade*, one of the progressive movements in obstetrics is to reverse the old custom of excluding the father from the lying-in room. The father's right to be present is nowadays accepted not only in régimes where some form of 'natural childbirth' is practised, but in quite conventional hospitals. The move to exclude the father seems to be a sacrifice of common sense to feminist ideology.

(iv) The *radical-feminist* ideal sees physicians relegated to the status of technicians. It is envisaged that they must un-learn their professional role and be prepared to act in the capacity of a stand-by to be called only when and if lay practices and folkways in obstetrics have run the mother into difficulties. According to Ruzek:

> Professionals must also co-operate with or at least tolerate, unorthodox practitioners (for example astrologers, lay midwives or herbalists) patients select as primary caregivers or as authorities on health matters.[23]

But Ruzek regretfully admits that, 'in some traditionalist feminist groups physicians are expected to pitch in and do some "shit work" – for example sterilizing instruments and mopping clinic floors. . . . It is hard enough, however, to get physicians to volunteer medical skills without asking for this much sharing'.[24] It might be easier, perhaps, to get responsible physicians to accept the burden of the 'shit work', than to make them acknowledge the authority of astrologers, untrained midwives and herbalists as 'primary caregivers'. It seems more likely that the ideal of the radical-feminists will remain simply that – an ideal.

Although the feminists' advocation of mothers taking a greater share of responsibility for their well-being, rather than delivering themselves as passive objects into the care of the medical profession, may make for less pain and trouble in labour, there is a danger that their political zeal for breaking the power of the medical profession, and of the trained midwives who are perceived as medical hench-women, may result in the baby being (metaphorically) thrown out with the bathwater. The parturient women may become pawns in a political struggle and their real welfare overlooked. The feminist writers advocate that women should educate themselves about the anatomy of their bodies and the physiology of their functions, but in this matter they seem to be quite unaware that this has been advocated for quite half a century by the (male) pioneers of obstetric analgesia and 'natural childbirth'. The feminists do not appear to be at all well-informed about what has been going on in the pioneer movements before about 1970. It is easy to imagine that one is advocating totally new methods simply through ignorance of past history.

A more realistic approach to the problems of the expectant mother retaining her autonomy whilst co-operating usefully with professionals is given by Fagerhaugh and Strauss in *Politics of Pain Management*.[25] These authors are aware of how present practices have grown out of historical trends in medicine, nursing, midwifery and changing public opinion. They write:

> The dominant practices of medical care and organization are under attack from the outside by women's movements, bioethics movements, counter-culture movements, and other health movements, as well as from the inside of the world of medicine itself by movements concerned with such issues as death and dying, community medicine and primary medicine. In addition there are various medical speciality and occupational specialty bases for further ideological differences which add to the politicization, both subtle and obvious, of the work within hospitals.[26]

They also recognize the power of family tradition, nowhere more

strong than in the conduct of childbearing, which overrides to some
degree all health education and temporary ideological indoctrination
of the individual member of the family. They illustrate it by the
following account of a staff resident who tried to calm down a
parturient woman who was screaming louder than he thought her
present state justified. The woman rounded on him, saying, 'Look, my
mother screamed like this, my grandmother screamed like this, my
sisters screamed like this, and I'm going to scream like this!'[27]

IS PAIN IN CHILDBIRTH NECESSARY?

In order to reach an understanding of what methods are available to
women to achieve a satisfactory labour without unnecessary pain, we
must take a broad and historical view of the situation. Indeed, we must
ask the question of whether or not pain is inevitable. In modern
Western society a proportion of women who have no special
anatomical peculiarity do not experience any pain at all while giving
birth. Velvovski[28] has estimated this lucky minority as being from 7 to
14 per cent of the parturient population. How can we explain this
pecularity? As it does not appear to relate to any special anatomical
features, we may suppose that it relates to some special features of
personality organization, which may be determined principally by
genetic factors, or by factors of upbringing and experience. The fact is
that we simply do not know, and little research has been done on the
problem. It is interesting that about the same percentage of the
population are able to go into a deep hypnotic trance, and can be
rendered (or can render themselves) analgesic to noxious stimuli by
appropriate hypnotic suggestion. As is well known, hypnosis can be
used in childbirth to produce analgesia, but deep-trance subjects do
not inevitably do better than women in a lighter trance, although
there is quite a strong association between measures of susceptibility
and measures of benefit, as shown in the review by Hilgard and
Hilgard.[29]

The puzzle is, then, whether the approximate 10 per cent of women
who experience no pain are the 'normal' ones (i.e. healthy and
functioning in a proper manner) and the other 90 per cent the product
of some cultural and individual psychological aberrations, or vice
versa. Earlier in this chapter, some anthropological evidence was
mentioned showing that women in less developed communities do not
necessarily experience easier labours than those in highly developed
communities, but it may be argued that in this late stage in the
development of human culture, *all* societies, no matter how relatively
primitive they may appear to anthropologists, possess a lengthy social
history which has taken them a long way from the condition of our

original anthropoid ancestors. It is instructive therefore to consider the evidence concerning pain in the parturition of other species of the higher mammals.

Other species have the great advantage that the heads of their young are not so large in comparison with the width of the birth canal, so there is less reason for tissue damage and consequent pain. According to Rivière and Chastrusse,[30] veterinary experts are by no means unanimous as to the extent that domestic animals suffer pain in giving birth, and of course we can have no sure knowledge about animals in the wild state. Some vets allege that large domestic animals such as cows and mares clearly suffer pain in giving birth, groaning and crying in the second stage of labour. If epidural anaesthesia is administered the animal ceases its cries, so presumably the cause of the cries is pain. Bitches also show signs of pain in giving birth, and here a significant observation has been made: those that have been brought up hardily seem to suffer far less than those that have been reared in soft conditions. Possibly a difference in the breed of dog as well as the conditions of its rearing is also involved. Observations of animals have led to the conclusion that during the first period of labour the uterine contractions are probably not painful, but that pain may come when the head passes through the pelvic ring.

It is possible to take the position that although giving birth is a perfectly normal physiological function, generally it gives rise to some pain in the higher placental mammals – and why not? It has been to the advantage of the higher mammals in the course of evolution to develop large brains and hence uncomfortably large skulls. Various factors have determined the size of the pelvis, and hence the width of the birth canal, but provided the ratio between the size of the skull and the pelvis does not occasion too high an incidence of maternal mortality or crippling, or of damaged neonates, the pain of the mother is not going to affect evolutionary trends which are otherwise advantageous to the species. The anomaly that some 10 per cent of women do not suffer pain although they have no special anatomical advantages, is quite unexplained. Now that we have discovered such interesting mechanisms as the endorphin system, and understand a very great deal more about pain mechanisms in general, it is possible that research will elucidate this puzzle. Certainly it gives us hope that we will learn more about the reduction of the pain of childbirth in the generality of women.

THE PSYCHOLOGICAL CONTROL OF PAIN IN CHILDBIRTH

It is important to realize that the methods of such obstetric pioneers as Dick Read, Velvovski, Lamaze and Vellay were developed in an era when the specificity theory of pain was dominant, and that they made assumptions about the nature of pain conductance which some would consider a little naïve today. It is to their credit, however, that through the force of empirical evidence they were able to realize the immense role that psychological factors play in the experience of pain in childbirth. The roots of the movement for 'natural childbirth' are to be found in the mesmeric movement of the nineteenth century which went into a partial eclipse at the end of the century. The pharmacological control of obstetric pain, inaugurated by James Simpson's use of chloroform, then gained great popularity. The early use of chloroform was replaced around the turn of the century, by an innovation introduced by two German doctors, Kronig and Gauss, known as 'twilight sleep'.[31] It consisted of hourly hypodermic injections of a mixture of scopolomine and morphine to keep the parturient woman in an analgesic daze during labour, which it inevitably prolonged; it also gave the baby a dose of drugs via the placental circulation. This practice was not discontinued until the 1930s.

THE READ METHOD

Grantly Dick Read first described his method in 1933 in his book *Natural Childbirth*.[32] Three further books were to follow. He related how he had been called to deliver a child in a poor district of London, and as was customary with him he offered the woman chloroform, but she refused it. Later, when the birth was completed, he asked her why she had not accepted the anaesthetic and she replied that the whole process had not hurt at all, and added, 'It wasn't meant to, was it, Doctor?' This question set him wondering whether childbirth was 'meant to' hurt or not, and he came round to deciding that it was not. The theory which he eventually worked out was broadly as follows.

Civilization has brought psychological influences to bear on women so that they have come to regard childbirth with anxiety. Such anxiety gives rise to muscular tensions which interfere with the natural operation of the womb and associated muscles and prevent them from expelling the baby in a normal manner. Such resistance and tension gives rise to pain because the womb responds to excessive tension with a pain reaction like any other over-stressed muscle. The three evils of fear, pain and tension are thus not normal to the natural process of parturition, but have been engendered in the expectant mother by expectations current in our society.

Read was a pioneer in two ways; first, although he accepted a specificity model for his neurology, he realized that the *interpretation* which the woman put on the initial feelings of uterine contraction was all-important. If she interpreted these feelings as the expected 'pain' then the sympathetic system of the body would be activated and produce a 'state of tension throughout the body which provides for an increase in muscular power'. Second, he advocated the use of learning techniques of muscular relaxation similar to those which Jacobson had described in his book *Progressive Relaxation*.[33] The methods Read advocated involved a pre-natal training which he regarded as having three functions: education, physiotherapy and psychotherapy. In this he is really the father of the régimes which are now practised in the majority of ante-natal clinics where the welfare of expectant mothers is taken seriously. Before Read's pioneer efforts, a brief health check was generally considered all that was necessary for ante-natal care.

The 'education' consisted of teaching expectant mothers the simple facts of anatomy and physiology related to conception, pregnancy and childbirth, instruction that was badly needed in the early 1930s when a great amount of ignorance was common. The 'physiotherapy' consisted of giving the expectant mothers training in controlled muscular relaxation, a technique which takes some time to master, and, as has been so forcefully argued in a recent book by Edmonston,[34] produces a state of hypnosis in suitably constituted people. During the birth process mothers were instructed to employ the relaxation methods they had learnt, at the point when they were informed that they had reached the stage of two-finger dilatation. In the expulsive phase the mother was expected to relax herself deeply between the strong uterine contractions.

Read was also a pioneer in his advocacy of the father's participation in obstetric care, and sensibly advised how he could lend practical as well as moral support, e.g. in massaging the lumbar region when required as an analgesic at the stage of complete dilatation. In the later development of his methods, Read placed great stress on proper breathing, as in his *Antenatal Illustrated*.[35] In this he simply follows in the tradition of Hatha Yoga.

Read's 'psychotherapy' was inherent in his total programme. He proceeded on the assumption that obstetric difficulty and pain were caused primarily by fear (by which he really meant anxiety), and he reasoned that with the woman's increased understanding of the process, and with acquisition of a greater control over her body reinforced by a trusting rapport with her physician, fear would be overcome and all desirable ends would follow. He realized that his psychotherapeutic programme involved strong suggestive influences, but for various reasons he did not care to admit that he was using a form of hypnosis and training his patients in auto-hypnosis. Experienced hypnotists such as Mandy[36] and Kroger,[37] when they came to examine Read's methods, were in no doubt at all that his methods depended largely on hypnotism. In fact, in describing his most successful cases, Read gives a good description of the behaviour of people in a somnambulistic state. Yet Read strongly resisted the assertion that he was doing very successfully what pioneer hypnotists such as Liébault, Bernheim and Bramwell had done before him. He wrote:

> I do not hesitate to record that so startling were the results of this teaching when I first employed it in the practice of natural childbirth, that I became suspicious of myself although I was aware that no conscious effort was being made to influence the minds of my patients by suggestion or hypnotism. Consequently I consulted one of the greatest authorities upon these subjects, and asked him to examine me and my methods to see whether by some accident I was unwittingly employing the use of methods of which I was unconscious. . . . I was assured that there was no relation whatever between the application of relaxation in obstetrics and strong suggestion, mesmerism or hypnotism.[38]

We are left wondering who the 'authority' was who gave so strange an assurance. In the 1953 edition of *Childbirth Without Fear* Read partly retracted his dogmatism on the subject in answer to Kroger's criticism.

Read attracted followers, including Helen Heardman, a physiotherapist who spread his methods in Britain, and Goodrich and Thoms who did the same in the USA. Today there is surely no developed country in the world where obstetric methods have not been influenced by Read. When controlled studies came to be done, often involving comparisons between thousands of mothers who had and had not been given the training for 'natural childbirth', it was found to the disappointment of many that the method neither shortened the labour nor reduced the incidence of lacerations and other obstetric complications. However, most of those who carried out the controlled studies[39] were prepared to agree that the mothers who had had the training showed less tension and anxiety, and, as they demanded less analgesics, presumably suffered less pain. It is quite clear, however, that Read's early hope that he could usher in an era of painless childbirth was to be disappointed. It is significant that the title of the American edition of his second book, published eleven years after his first, was *Childbirth Without Fear*.[40] Fear (or rather anxiety) could be banished more easily than pain.

THE RUSSIAN PSYCHOPROPHYLACTIC METHOD

This method, which has spread in Western Europe and America largely through the writings of the French obstetricians Lamaze and Vellay,[41] was derived quite deliberately from hypnotism, a branch of psychology which never suffered in Russia from the partial eclipse which affected it in the West. At a Leningrad conference in 1951, Nicolaiev stated that 'the roots of the Psychoprophylactic Method are found in our previous hypnosuggestive method based on Pavlov's doctrines'.[42] The Russians had experimented with hypnosis for twenty-five years and satisfied themselves that verbal suggestion could produce analgesia, and that it had no adverse effect on the new-born child. But as every hypnotist has found, all subjects are not equally susceptible to hypnosis however hard they try to co-operate, and the Russian obstetricians were seeking a technique which would be equally accessible to every doctor and midwife and could be applied on a national scale. The method they arrived at was basically similar to Read's in practice, but with a huge overload of Pavlovian theorizing to justify it. Russians seem to delight in theory for the sake of theory even more than do Western scientists, and although Velvovski and his colleagues were basically in agreement about the régime of ante-natal training that was introduced by the Ministry of Health of the Soviet Union in 1951, they by no means agreed among themselves as to how it should properly be justified in terms of Pavlovian physiology. By contrast, Read was rather naïve in his theory, and invoked the Freudian 'unconscious' to help explain his concepts. Various authors outside Russia have argued extensively as to the degree to which Read's methods and Russian Psychoprophylaxis are similar, and over the years the arguments have become rather sterile. The main difference would appear to be that Read put very great emphasis on muscular relaxation and thereby achieved a rather somnolent trance state in those mothers who were disposed to this sort of influence; the Russian method put more emphasis on alertness and active participation by the mothers, and continued to maintain the fiction that complete and utter painlessness could be achieved by everyone. The Russian scientists abandoned this fiction *among themselves* at the Kiev conference held after five years' experience with the method. It seems that the Russians aimed at producing the same sort of ideological exaltation which reached its peak in China at the height of the popularity of Chairman Mao, when patients would go into the operating theatre carrying the Red Book and endure a serious surgical operation with the aid of acupuncture alone. Such a state of exaltation can certainly achieve a remarkable degree of analgesia, but unfortunately not everyone has the temperament to attain it.

Paradoxically, while Read believed that his method was primarily a *psychological* one – the overcoming of fear – and used physical relaxation and breath control to achieve the psychological state of calm and indeed a hypnotic trance where possible, the Russians claimed that their method was basically *physiological*, stemming from the physiology of Pavlov, and injected into it a large element of ideological pep-talk and firm indoctrination that thoughts of pain were impermissible. In the contribution which he sent to a Paris symposium in 1957, Velvovski criticized Read for simply using hypnosis, and added:

> Fears and negative emotions are not for us the unique and determining cause of the pains. . . . We believe they rest upon the foundation of neurodynamic situations; they considerably increase unfavourable neurodynamic situations and complicate them.[43]

The history and the nature of the methods of Read and of Russian Psychoprophylaxis have been described at some length because the expectant mother who 'shops around' the various clinics will want to know just what the various contemporary ante-natal training regimes are based upon. Nowadays, Psychoprophylaxis is often referred to as the 'Lamaze Method' because it came to Britain largely through the efforts of Ferdinand Lamaze (who visited Russia in the 1950s and introduced the method to France). It does not matter greatly what the method is called, provided that adequate time is devoted to the training. Even if one understands the theory, it takes a good deal of practice to learn such a technique as controlled muscular relaxation, and it does not matter greatly whether the instructor is a midwife, physician, nurse, psychologist or physiotherapist. Many hospitals have their own versions of 'natural childbirth', and have introduced such useful innovations as group discussions with mothers who have already had their babies successfully with the method which is in vogue at the clinic.

HYPNOSIS IN MODERN OBSTETRIC PRACTICE
A good deal has already been explained about the use of hypnosis in overcoming pain. It is not necessary, therefore, to deal with this psychological technique in any great detail in relation to obstetrics. One advantage that hypnosis has over the other techniques which have been described is that it is more flexible and can be adapted more easily to the individual needs of the mother. If a woman is an adept at learning the techniques of self-hypnosis, after a few lessons she can put herself into an appropriate degree of trance and overcome unnecessary panic, tension and pain. It used to be thought that the hypnotic state is much more akin to 'sleep' (a somewhat ambiguous term, as we now realize) than we now know to be the case. Obstetric hypnotists had the erroneous idea that the hypnotized mother would undergo her labour not knowing what was taking place, and would remember nothing about it later. Greater knowledge of hypnosis has made it clear that the hypnotized mother knows perfectly well what is going on, and can direct her behaviour in a purposeful way. Afterwards she can

remember quite clearly all about the labour, although some people experience an oddly calm detachment in the manner illustrated by the reports of Chertok's two surgical patients described in Chapter 5. Part of the confusion about hypnosis is due to the fact that many doctors and lay people confuse it with mesmerism, and imagine that there will be an automatic post-hypnotic amnesia, a condition which is relatively rare when it has not been specifically suggested.

Both the Read method and Psychoprophylaxis involve quite a long period of ante-natal training beginning about eight weeks before the birth is due. This longish period of preparation is probably all to the good if the expectant mother needs to be educated in health matters concerning later pregnancy and childbirth when she has absolutely no prior knowledge. Although it is useful if ante-natal training in hypnosis is extended over a period, the skill can be learnt by some people relatively quickly; indeed hypnosis can be used without any ante-natal preparation at all. Thus Schibly and Aaronson[44] used obstetric hypnosis successfully with seventy-eight out of ninety-three unprepared women in a home for unmarried mothers (where presumably some had recently arrived), even carrying out some repairs of episiotomies with hypnotic analgesia alone. Whether or not the mother needs to have the attendance of a hypnotist at some time during the labour, will depend on the extent of her ante-natal training and on various other personal factors.

It is usual for the obstetrician-hypnotist to start with group hypnosis with small groups of expectant mothers, as this is greatly saving of time. Individual attention may later be given according to individual need. If possible, husbands should attend such sessions, for the more they become familiar with the whole process the better, and they may contribute useful help during the birth process. In ante-natal hypnosis actual rehearsal of the labour may be suggested and hallucinated in fantasy: Cheek and LeCron[45] use the hypnotic technique of suggesting that the mother projects herself forward in time and experiences a comfortable, successful labour, terminating in the welcome cries of the new-born baby. Obstetricians vary in their use of hypnosis as to whether it is directed primarily to control the delivery process and to determine the length of the different phases, or whether it is concentrated primarily on the production of analgesia. Thus Abramson and Heron,[46] working with one hundred women hypnotized individually, found that they could shorten both the first and second stages of labour, compared with a control group of seventy-eight women. By contrast, Cheek and LeCron, in the study cited above, concentrated on securing analgesia, suggesting, for instance, that the mother would feel herself 'numb from the waist down'. Whether this suggestion of a feeling of 'numbness' is altogether desirable, is debatable, for some people associate numbness with paralysis, and the parturient woman is to be encouraged to continue to make active movements to expel the baby, and later the after-birth. Posthypnotic suggestions of analgesia and comfort after the confinement is over are of course beneficial, and August[47] suggests that such suggestions may be used to promote early lactation.

When we turn to the published literature that might establish the extent to which hypnosis is a useful technique in obstetrics compared with other methods, the results are disappointing. Physicians who practise hypnosis are not often very scientifically oriented, and many of them try to preserve the medical myth that anyone can be hypnotized by doctors as gifted as themselves. In order to assess the usefulness of hypnosis, we have to know something about the varying degrees of hypnotic susceptibility among the women with whom the technique was used. If the technique has been a complete failure with some of the women in a study (as inevitably it will be) it is pointless to relate their degree of 'success' or 'failure' in labour (measured in terms of length, pain experienced, tissue damage, etc.) to any supposed hypnotic effect. Such an exercise is rather like trying to assess the efficacy of a certain drug in a population in which certain individuals have omitted to swallow the drug.

There are a number of very useful scales of hypnotic susceptibility which psychologists have devised as the result of a great deal of research, but few physicians will use them in clinical practice. An unusual, and unfortunately rather small study of the efficacy of hypnosis in obstetrics is that of Rock, Shipley and Campbell,[48] who tested twenty-two mothers on a rather simple scale of hypnotic susceptibility, and used the same hypnotic technique with all of them during labour. Comparing their report of experienced pain with that of a control group whom they did not attempt to hypnotize, the hypnotic technique was shown to reduce pain by a significant amount. This study also showed that within the group given the hypnotic treatment, those who scored higher on the scale of susceptibility tended to experience less pain.

Despite the lack of much available evidence, it seems safe to conclude four things. First, that hypnosis is useful in promoting analgesia in labour with many but not all women; second, that the mysterious fact of differential susceptibility to hypnosis among different individuals is relevant to the success of the method; third, that even if some individuals are quite insusceptible to hypnosis, they may benefit to some degree from the whole 'ritual' as a placebo, just as they may benefit from the magic of the name of Grantly Dick Read or Psychoprophylaxis or from a plaster statuette of a saint displayed in the labour ward; fourth, that, as noted by Velvovski and others, there is the baffling fact that from 7 to 14 per cent of parturient women will experience no pain at all for reasons which are entirely unknown. Given these four interacting variables, considered against a certain medical reluctance to engage in properly controlled research into clinical hypnosis, it is understandable that we cannot be more definite about the capacity of hypnosis, and other psychological techniques, to reduce pain in childbirth.

THE EPICUREAN TECHNIQUE

It has been suggested above that the endeavours of Cheek and LeCron to produce numbness from the waist down in parturient women, by hypnotic suggestion, may be ill-conceived because of the association which many people make between numbness and paralysis. An alternative approach is to leave the mother perfectly well aware of her sensations and movements, but to get her to experience what is happening as pleasure rather than pain. The immediate reaction to this suggestion of some women who have experienced extreme obstetric pain, or of midwives and others who have witnessed parturient women in pain, may be one of incredulity and even of scorn, but nevertheless it does make sense if viewed in the total context of female sexuality as expounded by Niles Newton.[49] Such a drastic reorientation of experiential responses implies a period of very special ante-natal training.

Niles Newton maintains that sexuality in the female is utterly different from male sexuality, and embraces the functions of copulation, parturition and breast-feeding, all of which are *potentially* pleasurable and closely linked. There are in fact a number of women (and Newton does not even attempt to guess at a percentage) who report that for them parturition was not just painless but positively ecstatic, involving a recognizable sexual experience culminating in orgasm. Masters and Johnson[50] reported on twelve women who described their experience of childbirth as being of this nature. Newton also mentions an obstetrician who noted that in some of his patients when the cervix was completely dilated there was a clitoral erection maintained until the birth was complete. She publishes a table listing eleven close similarities, physiological, behavioural, emotional, anatomical and sensory, which link undrugged childbirth with the experience of intercourse and orgasm in women.

(The fact that even when perineal tissue is being torn intense sexual pleasure can be experienced by the mother, may be repugnant to some people because they fear that, by a process of false reasoning, this may be used to bolster up the male fantasy that some women enjoy being raped. Let us stress, therefore, that enduring rape and enjoying one's own sexual functions are in no way comparable.)

We may search the obstetric literature in vain for any adequate discussion of this phenomenon or hard facts to clarify the issue. It seems that few women are willing to tell their doctors what a wonderfully sexy experience they have enjoyed during childbirth, and indeed, it seems likely that some of the cries, gasps and grimaces which doctors and midwives interpret as expressions of pain, may be the usual concomitants of orgasm. Contemporary views about pain, and about female sexuality, may not be flexible enough to conceptualize the phenomenon adequately. Contemporary feminist literature has tended to propagate a rather narrow and dogmatic view of female sexuality, basing it somewhat paradoxically on the model of male, phallic sexuality and hence over-stressing the role of the clitoris in orgasm. Some feminists argue very heatedly about what they refer to as 'the myth of the vaginal orgasm', as though there were only one possible means of achieving orgasm. However, more scientific studies of sexuality such as that of Kinsey et al.[51] have stressed the enormous inter-individual variability of sexual behaviour and experience. It seems not unreasonable to suppose that with some women sexuality involves the whole generative system, and that childbirth can trigger off the massive neural mechanisms of orgasm and pleasure.

This section is labelled 'The Epicurean Technique' because it is possible by hypnotic suggestion to oppose pain not by passivity and numbness but by the alternative means of developing imagery of activity and positive pleasure – not necessarily of a sexual nature. In other words, one rejects the negative Stoic philosophy of Zeno in favour of the positive philosophy of Epicurus. In the present instance this has been exemplified in relation to childbirth, where sexual imagery is indeed appropriate, but the Epicurean rationale can be applied to other conditions which are potentially painful. This theme will be developed in the next chapter.

Naturally there are some practical difficulties in introducing an expectant mother to the view that her coming confinement may be viewed in terms of a positive sexual experience. Women will vary very much as to the degree to which the coming experience can be eroticized in their expectation. Unquestionably, in the great majority of cases, the husband needs to be very closely involved in this exercise, but once the expectant mother can be persuaded intellectually to consider the proposition that childbirth can be an exciting and enjoyable culmination of her sex life, rather than a dreaded ordeal of pain, and her private sexual fantasies enhanced by training in auto-hypnosis, she may go a long way towards re-orienting her information processing system so that the massive neural stimuli arising from the event become experienced as pleasure rather than pain. Recognition of the existence of immense individual differences makes it evident that no therapist should attempt to direct an expectant mother as to *how* she should use her sexual fantasies; the woman is the best judge of that. What the therapist can do is to explain the possibilities of keeping childbirth within the domain of actively pleasurable sexual experience, and to help her master the techniques of auto-hypnosis to achieve this end.

REFERENCES

1 B. A. J. C. Gregory, 'The menstrual cycle and its disorders in psychiatric patients. I. Review of the literature', *Journal of Psychosomatic Research*, 1957, 2, pp. 61–79.

2 A. J. Coppen and N. Kessel, 'Menstruation and personality', *British Journal of Psychiatry*, 1963, 109, pp. 711–21.

3 E. Wittowker and A. T. M. Wilson, 'Dysmenorrhoea and sterility: personality studies', *British Medical Journal*, 1940, 2, pp. 586–90.

4 A. Broadhurst, 'Abnormal sexual behaviour – females', in H. J. Eysenck, (ed.), *Handbook of Abnormal Psychology*, London: Pitman, 1973.

5 P. Weideger, *Female Cycles*, London: The Women's Press, 1975.

6 S. B. Ruzek, *The Women's Health Movement*, New York: Praeger Publishers, 1978, p. 87.

7 G. Théano, 'The prevalence of menstrual symptoms in Spanish students', *British Journal of Psychiatry*, 1968, 114, pp. 271–3.

8 R. H. Moos, 'The development of a menstrual distress questionnaire', *Psychosomatic Medicine*, 1968, 30, pp. 853–67.

9 K. Dalton, *The Menstrual Cycle*, New York: Pantheon Books, 1969.

10 R. M. Dorcus and F. J. Kirkner, 'The use of hypnosis in the suppression of intractible pain', *Journal of Abnormal and Social Psychology*, 1948, 43, pp. 237–9.

11 F. G. Mullen, 'The treatment of a case of dysmenorrhoea by behaviour therapy techniques', *Journal of Nervous and Mental Disease*, 1968, 147, pp. 371–6.

12 W. E. Fordyce, *Behavioral Methods for Chronic Pain and Illness*, op. cit.

13 P. Weideger, *Female Cycles*, op. cit., pp. 242–3.

14 A. L. Kroeber, *Anthropology*, New York: Harcourt, 1948.

15 See W. H. Trethowan and M. F. Coulon, 'The couvade syndrome', *British Journal of Psychiatry*, 1965, 111, pp. 57–66.

16 L. Chertok, *Psychosomatic Methods in Painless Childbirth: History, Theory and Practice*, (Trans. D. Leigh), London: Pergamon, 1959.

17 L. Z. Freedman and V. M. Ferguson, 'The question of "painless childbirth" in primitive cultures', *American Journal of Orthopsychiatry*, 1950, 20, pp. 363–72.

18 S. B. Ruzek, *The Women's Health Movement*, op. cit.

19 S. Arms, *Immaculate Deception: A New Look at Women and Childbirth in America*, Boston: Houghton Mifflin, 1975.

20 G. J. Barker-Benfield, *The Horrors of the Half-known Life*, New York: Harper & Row, 1976.

21 M. Goodnow, *Nursing History*, Philadelphia; W. B. Saunders, 1958, p. 203.

22 S. B. Ruzek, *The Women's Health Movement*, op. cit., p. 108.

23 Ibid. p. 110.

24 Ibid.

25 S. Y. Fagerhaugh and A. Strauss, *Politics of Pain Management*, Memlo Park, Calif.: Addison-Wesley Publishing Co., 1977, p. v.

26 Ibid.

27 Ibid., p. 229.

28 I. Z. Velvovski, cited by L. Chertok, *Psychosomatic Methods in Painless Childbirth*, op. cit., p. 191.

29 E. R. Hilgard and J. R. Hilgard, *Hypnosis in the Relief of Pain*, op. cit.

30 M. Rivière and L. Chastrusse, 'La doleur en obstetrique', *Revue Français de Gynecologie et d'Obstetrique*, 1954, 49, pp. 247–76.

31 See H. A. Skinner, *The Origin of Medical Terms*, New York: Hafner Publishing Co., 1970, p. 413.

32 G. D. Read, *Natural Childbirth*, London: Heinemann, 1933.

33 E. Jacobson, *Progressive Relaxation*, Chicago: University of Chicago Press, 1929.

34 W. E. Edmonston, *Hypnosis and Relaxation*, New York: J. Wiley, 1981.

35 G. D. Read, *Antenatal Illustrated: The Natural Approach to Happy Motherhood*, London, Heinemann, 1957.

36 A. J. Mandy, R. Farcus, E. Scher and T. E. Mandy, 'The natural childbirth illusion', *Southern Medical Journal, Birmingham* (USA), 1951, 44, pp. 527–34.

37 W. S. Kroger, 'Natural childbirth: Is the Read Method of "Natural Childbirth" waking hypnosis?', *Medical Times*, 1952, 80, p. 152.

38 G. D. Read, *Revelation of Childbirth*, London: Heinemann, 1942, p. 165.

39 For early assessments of Read's methods see H. Roberts, L.T.D. Wooten, K. M. McKane and W. E. Hartnett, 'The value of ante-natal preparation', *Journal of Obstetrics and Gynaecology of the British Empire*, 1953, 60, pp. 404–8. Also: W. C. W. Nixon, 'Foreword', in H. Heardman, *Physiotherapy in Obstetrics and Gynaecology*, Edinburgh: E. & S. Livingstone, 1951.

40 G. D. Read, *Childbirth Without Fear*, New York: Harper, 1953.

41 F. Lamaze and P. Vellay, *Psychologic Analgesia in Obstetrics*, New York: Pergamon, 1957.

42 A. P. Nicolaiev, 'Conclusion', in *Leningrad Congress*, cited by L. Chertok, op. cit.

43 I. Z. Velvovski, cited by F. Lamaze and P. Vellay, op. cit.

44 W. J. Schibly and G. A. Aaronson, 'Hypnosis: Practical in obstetrics?' *Medical Times*, 1966, 94, pp. 340–3.

45 D. B. Cheek and L. M. LeCron, *Clinical Hypnotherapy*, New York: Grune & Stratton, 1968.

46 M. Abramson and W. T. Heron, 'An objective evaluation of hypnosis in obstetrics: Preliminary report', *American Journal of Obstetrics and Gynecology*, 1950, 59, pp. 1069–74.

47 R. V. August, *Hypnosis in Obstetrics*, New York: McGraw-Hill, 1961.

48 N. Rock, T. Shipley and C. Campbell, 'Hypnosis with untrained, non-volunteer patients in labour', *International Journal of Clinical and Experimental Hypnosis*, 1969, 17, pp. 25–36.

49 N. Newton, 'Trebly sensuous woman', *Psychology Today*, 1975, 1, pp. 34–8.

50 W. H. Masters and V. E. Johnson, *Human Sexual Response*, London: Churchill, 1966.

51 A. C. Kinsey, W. B. Pomeroy, C. E. Martin and P. H. Gebhard, *Sexual Behavior in the Human Female*, Philadelphia: Saunders, 1953.

9

COMING TO TERMS WITH PAIN

The Necessity for Pain

Acute pain is often referred to as 'nature's warning', and as is well known, we cannot do without it. The pain of a sudden prick, contusion or burn ensures that immediate action is taken to protect the injured part, and even less immediate pains are indispensable for the maintenance of health and for recovery from injury. An injured part will often ache, and the pain we experience ensures that sufficient attention is paid to the protection of that part during healing.

Recognition of the usefulness of acute pain has led to the formulation of the novel theory of Bolles and Fanselow[1] that pain can best be conceptualized as a 'motivational state of recuperation', as discussed in Chapter 4. Whether one accepts the theory or not, it seems reasonable to accept the general proposition that when physicians are confronted with a state of pain, they should first consider the diagnostic significance of the pain, and only later the question of relieving it.

Conditions of inability to experience pain are highly abnormal. They may be acquired and temporary, or congenital and longstanding. As was mentioned in Chapter 6, some conditions of schizophrenic disorder, regarded by many theoreticians such as Petrie[2] as conditions of extreme 'perceptual reduction', confer an astonishing immunity to pain. Conditions of conversion hysteria may bring on a temporary anaesthesia, typically to a local part of the body; temporary local anaesthesia may also follow from neural damage, as in the sequelae of a stroke.

The rare permanent conditions of inability to experience pain are less easily explained: they were commented on by Weir Mitchell[3] in 1892, and an extensive review of them was made fifty years later by Critchley.[4] Some of these conditions are congenital, and may be associated with severe mental subnormality, but many also occur in people of normal and high intelligence.

The possession of normal sensitivity to pain is therefore something which follows from a healthy adjustment to the environment. The mechanisms by which pain can be experienced to a greater or lesser degree according to the demands of the immediate situation, have been discussed in earlier chapters. While admitting that pain is an entirely necessary experience, it is natural that humans, who constantly seek greater and greater control over their environment, should strive for ways and means of coming to terms with pain, just as they must seek to come to terms with frustration, sorrow and the fact of their own mortality. What irks us is that some pain appears to be *unnecessary* and serves no function at all in keeping us in health and safety. This point has already been discussed in relation to chronic pain and women's pains, but it deserves further elucidation. Perhaps if we can come to terms with pain, although we may still have to experience it even when it is useless, we will not *suffer* as much, because suffering is very much bound up with our emotions and attitudes. Pain need not ruin our happiness and all enjoyment of life as a rewarding experience.

Pain as a Driving Force

It has been argued in this book that pain does two things: first, it *alerts* us to the fact that something is wrong, informing us of where in the body there is a threat to our integrity; second, it *compels* us to try to do something about it. It is this element of compulsion, the affective and motivational aspect of pain, which makes us feel that certain conditions are 'unbearable', that we cannot, will not, permit their continuance for another moment, and that all other considerations are overridden by the mastery of pain. Such a violently emotional and motivational state may come to dominate the whole life of the sufferer and break him down so that he acts quite out of character as though he were suffering from a severe mental illness. From his experiences in the American Civil War, Weir Mitchell commented that:

> Perhaps few persons who are not physicians can realize the influence which long-continued and unendurable pain may have upon both body and mind. . . . Under such torments the temper changes, the most amiable grow irritable, the soldier becomes a coward, and the strongest man is scarcely less nervous than the most hysterical girl.[5]

Intellectually we know that there is nothing further that we can do about the ache of a crushed limb, the nagging pain of a healing burn, or the slow progress of an inoperable tumour (apart from resorting to drugs or other artificial techniques), but as our primitive mechanisms of pain were developed long before the evolution of our intellectual capacity, we feel impelled to take some action. Our problem is to accept the inevitable and redundant content of the pain experience, and to negate the terrible urgency of the feeling that we must 'do something about it'.

Religious and Philosophic Views

The 'injustice' of pain which serves no useful function has prompted considerable speculation by religious writers and philosophers who are concerned with the goodness and intent of God in his creation of the universe. Why is pain visited upon the innocent, serving to warp rather than to ennoble the moral character? Why are some lives lived out in the misery of senseless pain when they are doomed to extinction anyway? Our modern technological age has at last supplied some partial remedies for these ugly facts, but what have religions and philosophers to say about their implications? In order to seek answers to these questions, we must take a broad approach to the problems, considering humanistic, religious and philosophical views such as impinge on us in Western culture. For although this book has been largely an inquiry into the nature of pain and how it may be conquered, its value will be limited if it does not also address issues of moral understanding and compassion which are in a somewhat different although related universe of discourse.

The Book of Job provides an outstanding commentary on the suffering of pain by the innocent. As St Thomas Aquinas noted of this Book, 'Nothing appears more to impugn divine providence in human affairs than the affliction of the innocent'.[6] The Book of Job provides a somewhat unusual indeed even heretical example of a Judaic view of pain, which is in itself rather different from the Christian view. In this dramatic poem, when the Sons of God present themselves before their Lord, Satan, who is among them, makes the philosophical point that piety, as exemplifed by Job, is merely the result of enjoying divine favour and worldly riches. The Lord accepts the challenge, and allows Satan to strip Job of all his goods and to kill his children. After this devastating act, Job still remains pious and does not fulfil Satan's prophecy that 'he will renounce thee to thy face'. Satan then goes further and proposes that whilst losing all one's goods and family is one thing, to be afflicted by sickness and pain is another, and that if Job were sorely afflicted in his physical body he would react to this totally unmerited pain by cursing his maker.

When the more severe trial is embarked upon, Job's three friends, who act as a chorus in the drama, present the conventional view of pain being necessarily a punishment for sin, and urge Job to search his conscience and repent. With growing fervour, Job then advances the argument that as he is totally guiltless he has nothing to repent; the remarkable fact emerges that his affliction is totally *unmerited*.

Although Job himself does not pass judgement, God is arraigned for acting contrary to justice. Soon Job is answered by the Voice out of the Whirlwind, which gives a magnificent panegyric on the wonders of the universe and the illegitimacy of comparing it with the pettiness of man's judgement, and indeed all human existence and experience. There is no answer that Job can make, for his sufferings are meaningless in terms of the greatness of cosmic forces.

The Book of Job has generally been interpreted as displaying a paragon of piety and patience to be emulated in adversity, but another interpretation is that its author was arguing the futility of seeking for some form of justification for pain and disaster in terms of an anthropomorphic concept of the deity, who was supposed by the ignorant to relate pains to their ideas of merit and sin.

Writers on religious topics in the Christian tradition have enlarged on the theme of unmerited pain in various ways. *The Problem of Pain* by C. S. Lewis[7] is remarkable for having run into twenty impressions in sixteen years, and therefore appears to have appealed to a very wide public. It should be noted that C. S. Lewis was not a theologian but a popular lay writer. Originally an atheist, he achieved a great following through his many religious books. In Lewis' view, 'We can rest contentedly in our sins and in our stupidities. . . . But pain insists upon being attended to. God whispers to us in our pleasures, speaks in our conscience, but shouts in our pains; it is his megaphone to arouse a deaf world'.[8]

In this Christian view, pain is God's remedy for sin, not the sin of disturbed social relations, but the sin of the pride of selfhood. But if we enquire how terrible pain can be deserved even by young children in cases where the pain serves no biological function, Lewis' view is that:

Such a sin requires no complex social relations, no extended experience, no great intellectual development. From the moment a creature becomes aware of God as God and of itself as self, the terrible alternative to choosing God or self for the centre is opened to it. This sin is committed daily by young children and ignorant peasants as well as by sophisticated persons.[9]

In essence, Lewis' view is that there is no unmerited pain; the young child as well as the sophisticated adult has deserved his suffering by virtue of his being human, and having therefore partaken of the guilt of Adam's fall.

A somewhat more humane view of the problem of pain is expressed by the philosopher and Nobel laureate Albert Camus in his great novel *The Plague*.[10] Here he contrasts the attitude of the atheist doctor Rieux and the Jesuit priest Father Paneloux. The latter takes an orthodox Jesuit view of pain and calamity, and when it is confirmed that the town is stricken with plague, and the gates in the walls are closed to insulate the townspeople from infecting the neighbouring countryside, Father Paneloux preaches an eloquent and impressive sermon in the Cathedral. He begins, 'Calamity has come upon you my brethren, and, my brethren, you deserved it', then enlarges on the subject of God punishing the townspeople, old and young, virtuous and wicked, for the general state of moral corruption in their corporate life. Someone remarks, rather shrewdly, that Father Paneloux is a great scholar living an intellectual life, and that were he a humble parish priest living in contact with the daily pains and sufferings of poor parishioners he would have known better than to have preached such high-flown stuff.

Later, Father Paneloux comes to work with Dr Rieux in the plague hospital, and together they witness the terrible and prolonged agony of a dying child. The doctor, inured though he is to the sight of suffering, is deeply distressed by this purposeless ordeal, and afterwards, remembering the priest's sermon, rounds on him declaring, 'Ah! That child, anyhow, was innocent – and you know it as well as I do!' Then follows a moving scene in which the priest, a man of deep sincerity, tries to comfort his distressed colleague, urging that the problem of pain is too great for human understanding, and that all we can do is to love. To this the doctor replies:

'No, Father. I've a very different idea of love. And until my dying day I shall refuse to love a scheme of things in which children are put to torture.'[11]

The Plague is an allegorical book concerned with more than the problems of sickness, pain and death; but its philosophical portrayal of moral dilemmas helps to elucidate the problems of coming to terms with the pain we must ourselves experience, and witness in those around us.

One might have expected the existentialist philosophers to have had quite a lot to say on the subject of coming to terms with pain, for they regard man's significance not according to what he has been in the past, but in terms of his present state and what he is becoming. Surprisingly, the psychological problem of continued pain has received scant attention either from the original religious existentialists such as Kierkegaard and Karl Jaspers, or from the modern atheist ones such as Jean-Paul Sartre. Although not absolutely disregarding the subject of coming to terms with pain (as contrasted with spiritual anxiety), in general the existentialists have little to offer us.

Abraham Maslow, identified by Davison and Neale[12] as having been one of the greatest American existentialist therapists, neglects the problems of pain almost entirely in his influential book *The Farther Reaches of Human Nature*,[13] although he has a great deal to say about the problems of living, mental and physical health.

The existential therapist tries to deal with reality not as he, the therapist, perceives it (i.e. the patient's objective condition), but in terms of the patient's subjective experience. This is naturally highly relevant to the subjective experience of pain, and makes the distinction between 'organic' and 'psychogenic' pain less meaningful. The fact is, that modern existentialist therapists have turned their attention almost exclusively to conditions of psychological distress, or 'neurosis' in the commonly accepted usage of the term. Thus Maddi[14] talks of 'existential neurosis' and concentrates on patients whose problems concern a feeling of the meaninglessness of life; he neglects the problems of those to whom life would be very meaningful and rewarding were they not racked with the pains of excruciating conditions such as arthritis. Certainly we can see the relevance of conditions identified as 'existential neurosis' to the problem of coming to terms with pain, for if life is full, demanding and worthwhile, even a very painful condition will not utterly dominate the scene to the same extent. But it is not necessarily justifiable to identify a condition of neurosis with a condition of pain: they may have totally different origins and significance even when existing coincidentally.

An exception to the general neglect of the problem of pain by existential therapists is that of Thomas Szasz, whom Maslow fails to mention among the many existential therapists discussed in his book, possibly because Szasz is highly identified with Sartre whom Maslow rejects. Szasz is a psychiatrist who has achieved a certain notoriety because of his extreme criticisms of his psychiatric colleagues, notably in his book *The Myth of Mental Illness*.[15] As we have mentioned earlier, he holds the view that some people 'elect' to assume the full-time role expressed in Latin as *homini dolorosi*, that is, 'men of pain'. Such people suffer constant pain and allegedly use it as a basic means of communication with other people. According to Szasz:

> One thing strikes the careful observer of patients with chronic pain, especially in cases without organic illness: it is that they are individuals who have made a career of suffering. At one time such

persons may have been attorneys or architects, busboys or businessmen, models or maids; but when their careers fail or no longer suffice to sustain them, they become 'painful persons'; or to paraphrase the French diagnostic term *tic douloureux*, they become *hommes douloureux*. . . .[16]

(It should be noted that Szasz makes the assumption that chronic sufferers from pain have elected to adopt this strange career *because* their previous professions or trades have failed to satisfy them. Nowhere has he, or anyone else, advanced evidence to support this contention. Naturally, an injury or disease which sets off a condition of chronic pain, may disrupt or terminate a person's career however successful it may have been. It is another matter to impute career failure *post hoc* to those who have been so unfortunate. Certainly some remarkable people have continued successfully to pursue their careers despite conditions of chronic pain, but not all of us are so hardy, or cushioned by affluence, to attain this ideal.)

The concept of the patient embarking on a career of pain, accords to some degree with the views of Fordyce and his colleagues who have suggested that in some cases a painful way of life may be learned, and may thus persist after the original organic condition has cleared up. But as has also been pointed out, the *apparent* absence of an on-going organic condition which amply justifies the continuing pain may reflect more on the diagnostic competence of those caring for the patient than on actual reality. If it should eventually be discovered that a person who is presumed to be pursuing the career of *homo dolorosus* merely suffers from an improperly diagnosed condition that, say, a simple surgical operation will put right, such an operation will abruptly put an end to this presumed existentialist choice. Examples of simple organic conditions being overlooked, and misdiagnosis of psychogenic pain, are occasionally published in the medical press.[17] Because of such cases, dynamic psychiatrists might be presumed to be somewhat abashed when their elaborate hypotheses are demolished by a few strokes of the scalpel, but in general this is not the case, for dynamic psychiatry has its own defences which come into play in such eventualities.

But if indeed there are certain cases of pain patients about whom all that Szasz says is true, how does he propose to treat them? He points out that when faced with a 'painful person' the psychiatrist must choose between several courses. He may 'refuse to accept him as a patient' (a refusal hardly in keeping with the medical ethos, at least under the British NHS); he may undertake to treat him 'despite the patient's apparent desire to retain his painful identity'; or, having accepted him for treatment, he may 'insist that the patient choose whether he remain as he is or change'. Presumably, if the patient says that he 'chooses' to lose his pain, but still continues to suffer as much as he did at the beginning of treatment, then he is proven to be a humbug – for how else can Szasz retain his professional integrity?

Szasz quotes Sartre to the effect that:

> The social and material relation (between doctor and patient) is affirmed in practice as a bond even more intimate than the sexual act; but this intimacy is realized only by activities, and precise, original techniques engaging both persons. . . . Doctor and patient form a couple united by a common enterprise.[18]

If we accept this concept of the doctor-patient relationship, then it is as legitimate for the patient to accuse the doctor of 'choosing' that the pain shall continue and wilfully refusing to acknowledge or initiate measures that will lead to the termination of their intimate bond, as vice versa. After all, it is the patient who pays the doctor, directly or indirectly.

Practical Techniques

By mentioning the question of misdiagnosis and the problems arising therefrom, it is not implied that the generality of medical science is either incompetent in diagnostic skill or backward in seeking progress. The growing importance of the International Association for the Study of Pain, which incorporates so many medical and other specialists, attests to the rapid progress that is now being made in the conquest of pain. Neither is it implied that psychiatry as a whole is seeking to advance its frontiers within the medical profession at the expense of the occasional casualties of misdiagnosis. But what must be pointed out here is that the extreme existentialist fringe of psychiatry, which by some perversion of language is sometimes known as 'humanistic', wields a disproportionate influence with many members of the minor helping professions who deal with some pain patients, who do not appreciate that Szasz's portrayal of the bulk of his medical and psychiatric colleagues is a mere caricature.

The sufferer from long-continued pain, and those who are emotionally close to him, can accept the physician, nurse or other professional who frankly acknowledges that he simply does not know for certain what is causing the pain, and that the chance of an adequate diagnosis and effective remedy for the condition is not very good in the present state of knowledge. Such news is unwelcome, but the sufferer can feel that the best is being done for him in the circumstances. If, however, the physician or others tries to convince the patient that he knows very well what the trouble is – that he himself has 'chosen', out of moral weakness, perversity or deep dynamic conflicts, to become a pain patient, then there is a likelihood that the sufferer will develop a deep and brooding anger directed against those who attribute his sufferings to an existentialist choice. Such anger may greatly magnify his experience of pain. Alternatively he may relapse into a self-blaming depression, which is not only a powerful generator of additional pain, but may even lead him along the road of despair and suicide.

It is not only blame-shifting psychiatrists and their adherents who can engender this anger and despair in long-term sufferers from pain. Professor Wilkes of the University of Sheffield has recently castigated the

> . . . doctors who tend to wear white coats and to go around in small flocks like supercilious sheep, and who can only rarely and atypically be persuaded to sit on the bed and to talk patiently and frankly about the problems the patient is facing among all the expensive clutter and the teamwork of modern medicine and yet, so often, heartbreakingly alone.[19]

In the experience of the present writer, who has spent his share of time as a patient in hospital wards, one of the greatest advances in medicine in recent years has been that these 'supercilious sheep' are giving place to human beings, perhaps because they are more truly competent at their jobs, and therefore more ready openly to discuss the limitations of their knowledge. The great experts in the field of pain research, many of whom have been cited in this book, are characterized not only by their wide experience, their great learning and bold and original thinking, but by their true humility which acknowledges that the continued suffering of humanity from needless pain is a measure of the extent to which they and their sciences still fall short of their ideals.

Much evidence has been offered in this book that anger and depression enhances the experience of pain, and some writers such as Eisenbud[20] and Weiss[21] have suggested that it is the *suppression* of long-continued anger which exacerbates conditions of pain. Engel,[22] taking a rather more psychoanalytic view of the problem, suggests that the pain is exacerbated by guilt over hostility towards figures of power, which the sufferer dares not give vent to. Unfortunately these theories are mostly based on anecdotal clinical evidence rather than on controlled experimental research. It does seem inherently plausible, however, that the patient who regards himself as being negligently and incompetently treated will suffer all the more acutely if he is afraid to have the matter out with such powerful figures who protect themselves with professional arrogance. Many sufferers from recurrent conditions of pain, like migraine, readily admit that suppressed anger will bring on a painful attack, and indeed, Marcuson and Wolff[23] demonstrated that headache could be induced by inciting anger.

The general implications which arise from these studies of suppressed anger are similar to those which come from the 'learned helplessness' researches of Seligman.[24] In coming to terms with conditions which may generate pain the sufferer should retain as much autonomy over his own affairs as possible, and *not* seek to emulate the patience of Job. It is perfectly natural that those who have the care of pain patients should seek to encourage the saintly smile, and to pretend that suffering is an ennobling experience; but anyone who acts out of character and tries to pretend to be ennobled by pain, runs the risk of building up a reservoir of suppressed anger and hostility which will worsen the pain and sour his character.

Set against the dangers of suppressed anger and enforced humility is that of reverting to temper tantrums to get one's own way in all things, of becoming a dedicated pain patient, and thereby reinforcing the chronicity of the condition. Although the task of the helmsman is not an easy one, one must try to steer a middle course.

It is possible to introduce people to strategies for coming to terms with pain at any age, but the success with which they will attain this desired end must, to some degree, depend on the whole of their life's experience. If they have grown up expecting to swallow two or three pills every time they have a stomach-ache, and expect their GP to guarantee a pain-free existence, they are unlikely to develop adequate resistances to conditions which do not seriously incommode those individuals who are on more familiar terms with pain.

The relevance of general familiarity with pain to the later experience of its degree of intensity, is illustrated by a rather remarkable study recently carried out by Gerrard.[25] This study was designed to assess the nature and intensity of labour pain experienced by twenty-nine women. These mothers completed the McGill Pain Questionnaire (MPQ)[26] during the first stage of labour, and then repeated it post-natally in terms of their recent memory for the pain of the whole experience. As expected, the degree of pain experienced varied greatly between individuals; the results, however, came as a surprise to the investigator who had expected them to accord with a general theory of differential 'pain-proneness'. On the contrary, while physiological factors accounted for some of the differences, they were found to relate to another inquiry she conducted with the mothers concerning their past familiarity with pains unrelated to childbirth. Those women who had suffered from various sorts of pain during their previous life experience found that they suffered *less* in childbirth than those who had led comparatively pain-free lives. This contrast was quite clear and statistically significant in the study, and Gerrard, in discussing her results, suggests that it may be due to both psychological and physiological factors, the latter possibly depending on the development of the endorphin-secreting system as a well-established mechanism for coping with pain. Gerrard's study is very recent and as yet lacks confirmation by other researchers in obstetric pain related to past experience. It is possible, without straining the analogy too far, to relate it to the findings noted by Rivière and Chastrusse[27] that bitches accustomed to a relatively rough upbringing appear to experience very little pain in giving birth to their puppies, in contrast to those which have been more gently reared.

The general issue of how the NHS in Britain may contribute insidiously to increase the vulnerability of those it is designed to serve is discussed most intelligently and humanely by Andrew Malleson in *Need Your Doctor Be So Useless?*,[28] a book which should be on the shelves of all general practitioners and many patients. Malleson is not concerned specifically with the problems of pain, for his thesis is more general, but all that he writes is relevant to many of the issues which have been discussed in this book. He is not, of course, opposed to the sensible prescription of drugs for the alleviation of pain, but he inveighs against the staggering quantities of pills which are nowadays prescribed quite pointlessly. Again, whilst recognizing the enormous part that sympathetic and personalized care can play in maintaining people in health and combating sickness, he is strongly opposed to what he calls the element of impersonal 'baby care' that adults may come to accept as the norm. Some doctors tend to encourage an attitude of passive dependency in their patients, and reinforce it with a tremendous over-prescription of pills. People growing up in this climate of 'baby care' are hampered in developing an ability to come to terms with pain and ill-health, and to develop the robustness necessary to withstand the shocks and hazards of everyday life. The handing-out of 'baby care' is not at all incompatible with preserving the attitude of the white-coated 'supercilious sheep' which has aroused Professor Wilkes' anger. A few minutes of intelligent discussion and humanely expressed concern are worth bottles of analgesic pills and tranquillizers.

Although past experience is highly relevant to our present and future susceptibility to pain, some individual differences in suffering are related to personality factors, as has been discussed in Chapter 6. To some degree we are just 'born that way'. It follows that for the development of a robust and healthy resistance to pain, both in the upbringing of our children and in the management of our own affairs, we should use techniques which accord with our various innate personality traits. Those people who have an active and determined temperament and a dynamic drive to high achievement may suffer more from the conditions which generate 'useless pain' than those who are more apathetic and lethargic, for the former type are faced with a challenge which cannot properly be met. The motivational-affective component of their pain is generally high, and they may become so obsessed with seeking some meaning in their pain that eventually the pain becomes more of an 'emotional' than a 'physical' problem, and it is very greatly enhanced by frustration. For them, what is needed is development towards a more easy-going and extraverted attitude to life. But for everyone who has to give up work because of conditions of pain there is a need to return to some form of meaningful work just as soon as possible.

Whatever the innate temperament of an individual, no one should feel that he is doomed by his temperament to suffer from unnecessary pain. The healthiest psychological attitude for the pain-patient to cultivate is one of continued hope that his own efforts will eventually minimize and overcome the pain. There is also the very real hope that the steady progress of scientific research will eventually provide new techniques and remedies.

The story of the development of effective anaesthesia was not included in this book out of mere academic interest, but to make the point that pain *has* been conquered to a very great extent, that advances have been made, and will continue to be made, which would have seemed beyond the wildest hopes of two centuries ago. Science progresses, but each of us must make our own personal contribution to the conquest of pain, and if we ourselves suffer or have care of those who suffer, we must be prepared to fight, fight and fight again, in the sure knowledge that no physician, psychologist or other acknowledged 'expert' is the final authority on the private experience of a person's pain, or in prognosis for its future. Study of past history cuts the experts of every age down to size. Hope deferred need not make the heart sick: there is always hope in the conquest of pain, and in the achievement of personal happiness in spite of it.

The Epicurean Approach

At the end of Chapter 8 we mentioned briefly a form of therapy for pain derived from the philosophy of Epicurus. Although discussed there in terms of antenatal preparation, this approach is appropriate for all forms of pain, as well as for conditions of anxiety.

Two traditions have come down to us from ancient Greece: the Stoic philosophy associated with the name of Zeno, and the Epicurean philosophy associated with Epicurus. The words 'Stoic' and 'Epicurean' are part of our language, but the common meaning of them has suffered somewhat in usage, particularly because of later associations with Roman philosophy. In Rome, Stoicism came to be associated with the military code and extreme worship of the state; Epicureanism lost its higher associations and came to imply a gross sensualism. In their original Greek form, however, both were philosophies for attaining 'virtue', a concept of a well-ordered, healthy and happy life. Both stemmed from the older roots of Aristotelian philosophy, but whereas the Stoics taught a form of moral heroism and saw virtue residing in the ideal of the passionless sage, the Epicureans regarded pleasure and pain as the practical tests of virtue in all matters. Epicurus conceived the greatest good to be simple happiness, and happiness to be found in pleasure, to which the natural impulses of all healthy beings are directed. He differed slightly from the rather older school of the Cyrenaics (who emphasized the pleasure of the moment) by stressing the necessity for an enduring condition of pleasure, and regarding pain as the greatest of evils.

The Stoics dealt with the problem of pain by ignoring it; in their view the perfect sage would be theoretically immune to pain. The Epicureans admitted that on occasion the renunciation of pleasure or the voluntary endurance of pain might be a sensible means of ensuring a greater or more enduring pleasure. In Epicurean philosophy virtue was not conceived of as some nebulous value to be sought after for its own sake, but something to be sought for the sake of experiencing pleasure. Pleasure, in Epicurean terms, meant not just simple animal sensuality, but also the pleasure of the 'soul' (a concept which comes near to our modern concept of mind) and freedom from pain and fear.

The philosophy of Epicurus coincided with that of Zeno on many points, but it was rather more down to earth. They both agreed that the cardinal virtue was wisdom, but Epicurus held that wisdom was valuable only because it enabled us to calculate the consequences of our actions in terms of pleasure and pain. The Epicureans held that the pleasures of sense are subordinate to the pleasures of soul, or in other words that the mental pleasures of art, music, scientific endeavour and human love in its highest sense are a higher good than ephemeral sensuality or the freedom of the body from pain. The essential truth of this latter statement may be tested if we try to recall occasions on which we have been in a condition of physical well-being but in mental torture, and compare them with other occasions on which we have been in considerable pain but otherwise rather happy and at mental peace.

All our discussion of the nature of pain has indicated its great complexity, its blending of physical sensation with emotion and conative drive. But discussions of pleasure also reveal a similar complexity. The historical study of attitudes to pain, and attempts to control it, has revealed how much the Stoic philosophy has been taken for granted in Christian civilization. Pain has been opposed by grim resignation, the inculcation of numbness and literal insensibility brought on by drugs or other means. The Epicurean approach of opposing pain with positive feelings of pleasure has played a relatively small part in our history. Superficially, the latter idea seems unreasonable, for who, writhing in the throes of pain, can contemplate enjoyment of physical or mental delights? Yet the idea is neither unreasonable nor entirely original. The common-sense experience of mothers demonstrates that a lollipop is a fine analgesic for the painful contusions of childhood. Robert Burton[29] relates how some of the 'looser' physicians of his time would provide 'a beautiful young wench' as a remedy against pain, together with 'a potion or two of good drink'. Arthur Grimble[30] tells of a similar practice he encountered in the Solomon Islands, where the pain incidental to the long-continued ordeal of being extensively tattooed was assuaged by the affectionate embraces of two young maidens.

It has been described how some of the early analgesics and anaesthetics such as alcohol, nitrous oxide and ether were first used for their pleasure-giving properties, and not to deaden pain: indulgence in many drugs of abuse such as heroin is prompted initially by a quest for pleasure rather than for relief from pain. We are too apt to think of analgesia simply as a matter of 'deadening' pain.

At the level of laboratory experimentation and classroom demonstration it can easily be shown that pleasurable fantasy can inhibit or abolish pain. We have already described how Barber[31] had student nurses listen to a tape-recorded account of the alleged erotic adventures of a film star, whilst submitting to a mildly painful laboratory procedure, and it was shown that the pleasurable fantasies engendered had an analgesic effect. Similarly, a classroom demonstration of hypnotically-induced analgesia shows the same basic effect.[32] A hypnotized volunteer subject has it suggested to him that he is kissing someone whom he finds very attractive. When the actuality of the fantasy is manifested by the observed erection of the lips, he is asked to brush the back of his hand to and fro across his mouth, being assured that the warm, erotic glow of his lips will spread to his hand, and that the latter will take on a glow of pleasure and become enveloped, as it were, in a magic glove which transforms all sensations to pleasure. The hypnotist then asks the subject, whose eyes are closed, to fantasize something like the blade of a sword, assuring him that this blade could be passed through his protected hand without causing pain or injury, and that he would only experience pleasure. If permission is granted (as it generally is) the hypnotist then thrusts a surgical micro-lance through a substantial skinfold on the back of the hand. Afterwards, subjects report feeling no pain, and if the micro-lance is left *in situ*, the subject may be astonished to see it sticking in the back of his hand when he is aroused from the trance, as he has assumed that everything that has occurred was simply a pleasant hypnotic fantasy.

This demonstration is mentioned because it contrasts with an alternative means of achieving hypnotic analgesia of the hand by hypnotic suggestion. In the alternative method, the hypnotized subject is persuaded that his hand will become completely numb, perhaps by the fantasied injection of a local anaesthetic.[33] The objective result is the same, as an otherwise painful procedure may be carried out without hurting the hand, but the two methods illustrate the contrast between the Epicurean and the Stoic approach to achieving analgesia.

Not only can pain be overcome by opposing it with positive pleasure, but so also can anxiety. A great deal of behaviour therapy, much of it stemming from the original work of Wolpe,[34] depends upon controlling the patient's level of anxiety whilst presenting, in fantasy or reality, the objects, situations and ideas which form the basis of his phobias, obsessions and neurotic maladjustments. The most usual method of controlling the level of anxiety is to teach the patient to relax deeply, because according to Wolpe's theory of 'reciprocal inhibition', he will either be anxious, with tensed-up muscles, or relaxed and calm, with a relaxed musculature. This relaxation technique, which, as most dentists know, can also be used for the inhibition of pain, is a utilization of the approach that we have referred to as Stoic, for it opposes distress and pain with calmness, quiescence and non-response. But within behaviour therapy there is also a minor thread of the Epicurean approach, as the famous early study of Mary Cover Jones[35] in which one of the techniques for overcoming the phobia of a little boy for rabbits and similar furry objects was to feed him with chocolate whilst the feared object was being brought gradually nearer to him.

It is not suggested that the terrible problems of overcoming severe acute and chronic pains which some of us face can be achieved at the level of offering a child chocolate or engendering minor erotic fantasies. These examples have been quoted merely to illustrate the nature of the Epicurean approach. While much of conventional behaviour therapy stresses relaxation and non-feeling, as in the Grantly Dick Read preparation for childbirth, the alternative approach is to accept activity and to encourage arousal and powerful feelings, but to learn to process them so that they are experienced as pleasurable rather than painful. The belief that Epicureanism is merely concerned with trivial sensuality is misleading. Everyone knows the major sources of satisfaction in his own life; usually they entail intensive activity, mental or physical. Through such activity and what is for us high endeavour, we can come to terms with pain. The major problem is how to develop new sources of satisfaction when injury, disease or the usual processes of ageing reduce our previous avenues to fulfilment; but if we are perfectly clear as to the nature of the problem we can set about solving it in our own individual way.

For Whom the Bell Tolls

This book is written for a wide readership; those whose profession and dedication it is to help solve the problems of pain, those who are themselves in pain, and those who are at present in the best of health and well-being, but hear the tolling of the distant bell.

The era we have entered is unique in history. Never before has scientific technology been applied to health on the scale that it is today. Paradoxically, however, this has had the profound effect of making large numbers of us potential sufferers from chronic pain. In previous ages people died when they were young or middle-aged through a variety of acute illnesses and accidents, as is still the case in the 'Third World'. In the West today, thanks mainly to measures that we vaguely classify as 'public health', very many of us live on into old age. And as we grow older we tend to encounter the various degenerative diseases which, before causing death, may lead to years of suffering during which medical science keeps the sufferer alive without being able to protect him from pain. In this condition, the seventh age of man so graphically described by Shakespeare, we risk coming face to face with continued pain. At this time of life more than any other, psychological factors determine whether we shall drag out a miserable and painful existence, or live pleasantly, adapting to our fading faculties until we reach a quiet death.

What remedy, what philosophy can be advanced to meet the challenge that is before us, young and old? I can do no better than to quote the words of the great musician Pablo Casals, written at the age of ninety-three:

> On my last birthday I was ninety-three years old. That is not young of course. . . . But age is a relative matter. If you continue to work and to absorb the beauty in the world about you, you find that age does not necessarily mean getting old. At least, not in the ordinary sense. I feel many things more intensely than before, and for me life grows more fascinating. . . .
>
> Work helps prevent one from getting old. I, for one, cannot dream of retiring. Not now or ever. Retire? The word is alien and the idea

inconceivable to me. My work is my life. I cannot think of one without the other. To 'retire' means to me to begin to die. The man who works and is never bored is never old. Work and interest in worthwhile things are the best remedy for age. Each day I am reborn. Each day I must begin again.[36]

REFERENCES

1 R. C. Bolles and M. C. Fanselow, 'A perceptual-defensive-recuperative model of fear and pain', op. cit.

2 A. Petrie, *Individual Differences in Pain and Suffering*, op. cit.

3 S. Weir Mitchell, 'Precision in the treatment of chronic diseases', *Medical Record*, 1892, 42, pp. 721-6.

4 M. Critchley, 'Congenital indifference to pain', *Annals of Internal Medicine*, 156, 45, pp. 737-47.

5 S. Weir Mitchell, *Injuries of Nerves and Their Consequences*, op. cit.

6 St Thomas Aquinas, 'Prologue', *Summa Theologiae*.

7 C. S. Lewis, *The Problem of Pain*, London: Geoffrey Bles, 1956.

8 Ibid., p. 81.

9 Ibid., p. 63.

10 A. Camus, *The Plague*, Collected Fiction of A. Camus, London: Hamish Hamilton, 1970.

11 Ibid., p. 179.

12 G. C. Davison and J. M. Neale, *Abnormal Psychology*, New York: J. Wiley, 1974, p. 467.

13 A. H. Maslow, *The Farther Reaches of Human Nature*, Harmondsworth: Penguin Books, 1973.

14 S. R. Maddi, 'The existential neurosis', *Journal of Abnormal Psychology*, 1967, 72, pp. 311-25.

15 T. S. Szasz, *The Myth of Mental Illness*, London: Paladin, 1972.

16 Idem., 'A psychiatric perspective on pain and its control,' op. cit.

17 See J. Katz, 'Pain: theory and management', in C. Scurr and S. Feldman (eds), *Scientific Foundations of Anaesthesia*, London: Heinemann, 1970.

18 J. P. Sartre quoted by T. S. Szasz in 'A psychiatric perspective on pain and its control', op. cit. p. 47.

19 E. Wilkes, 'Doctors and the dying patient', in A. W. Harcus, R. Smith and B. Whittle (eds), *Pain: New Perspectives in Measurement and Management*, Edinburgh: Churchill-Livingstone, 1977, p. 132.

20 J. Eisenbud, 'The psychology of headache', *Psychiatric Quarterly*, 1937, 11, pp. 592-619.

21 E. Weiss, 'Psychogenic rheumatism', *Annals of Internal Medicine*, 1947, 26, pp. 890-900.

22 G. L. Engel, 'Primary atypical facial neuralgia: an hysterical conversion symptom', *Psychosomatic Medicine*, 1951, 13, pp. 375-96.

23 R. M. Marcuson and H. G. Wolff, 'A formulation of the dynamics of the migraine attack', *Psychosomatic Medicine*, 1949, 11, pp. 251-6.

24 M. E. P. Seligman, 'Depression and learned helplessness', op. cit.

25 C. Gerrard, 'A study of labour pain using the McGill Pain Questionnaire', unpublished study, 1981.

26 R. Melzack, 'The McGill Pain Questionnaire: Major properties and scoring methods', *Pain*, 1, pp. 277-99.

27 M. Rivière and L. Chastrusse, 'La doleur en obstetrique', op. cit.

28 A. Malleson, *Need Your Doctor Be So Useless?*, London: George Allen & Unwin, 1973.

29 R. Burton, *The Anatomy of Melancholy*, 1651.

30 A. Grimble, *A Pattern of Islands*, London: John Murray, 1954.

31 See T. X. Barber, 'Effects of hypnotic induction, suggestions of anesthesia, and distraction on subjective and physiological responses to pain', op. cit.

32 See H. B. Gibson, 'Pain mechanisms and their inhibition by hypnosis: The Epicurean Technique', Paper delivered in the British Society of Experimental and Clinical Hypnosis, Whittington Hospital, March 1980.

33 See T. X. Barber, N. P. Spanos and J. F. Chaves, op. cit., p. 26.

34 J. Wolpe, *Psychotherapy by Reciprocal Inhibition*, Stanford, Calif.: Stanford University Press, 1958.

35 M. C. Jones, 'The elimination of children's fears', *Journal of Experimental Psychology*, 1920, pp. 1-4.

36 A. E. Kahn (ed.) *Joys and Sorrows: Reflections by Pablo Casals*, New York: Simon & Schuster, 1970, pp. 15-17.

APPENDIX I

Speciality Areas Represented in the International Association for the Study of Pain

Behavioural sciences

Hypnosis
Neuropsychiatry
Neuropsychology
Neuropsychopharmacology
Physiological Psychology
Psychiatry
Psychoanalysis
Psychobiology
Psychology
Psychopharmacology
Psychophysiology
Psychosocial Rehabilitation
Psychosomatic Medicine
Psychotherapy
Sociology

Neural sciences

Neuroanatomy
Neurobiochemistry
Neurobiology
Neurochemistry
Neurocytology
Neuroendocrinology
Neuropathology
Neuropharmacology
Neurophysiology

Other basic sciences

Anatomy
Biochemistry
Bioengineering
Biology
Biometry
Comparative Physiology

Clinical sciences

Acupuncture
Allergy
Anaesthesiology
Community Health Education
Dentistry
Dental Prosthesis
Electromyography
Electroencephalography
Emergency Medicine
Endodontics
Family Practice
Gastroenterology
Haemorrhageology
Internal Medicine
Intensive Care
Neurology
Neuroprosthesis
Neuroradiology
Neurosurgery
Nursing
Obstetrics & Gynaecology
Occupational Therapy
Oncology
Ophthalmology
Oral & Maxillofacial Surgery
Orthopaedic Surgery
Pain
Periodontics
Perioral Pain
Pharmacology
Physiotherapy
Prostodontics
Radiation Therapy
Rehabilitation Medicine
Rheumatology
Spinal Cord Injury

Behavioural Sciences contd.

Cytology
Electrophysiology
Oral Biology/Physiology
Physiology
Toxicology

Other

History of Medicine
Research Administration
Public Information Specialist
Science Editor
Affiliates

Clinical sciences contd.

Stereoencephalotomy
Surgery
TMJ Dysfunction
Traumatology
Urology

From: J. J. Bonica and D. G. Albe-Fessard (eds), *Advances in Pain Research and Therapy*, New York: Raven Press, 1976.

APPENDIX 2

McGill - Melzack Pain Questionnaire

Patient's Name_____ Date_____ Time_____ am/pm
Analgesic(s) _____ Dosage_____ Time Given _____ am/pm
_____ .Dosage_____ Time Given_____ am/pm

Analgesic Time Difference (hours): +4 +1 +2 +3

PRI: S_____ A_____ E_____ M(S)_____ M(AE)_____ M(T)_____ PRI(T)____
    (1-10)   (11-15)   (16)   (17-19)   (20)   (17-20)   (1-20)

1 FLICKERING ___	11 TIRING ___	PPI_____ COMMENTS:
QUIVERING ___	EXHAUSTING ___	
PULSING ___	12 SICKENING ___	
THROBBING ___	SUFFOCATING ___	
BEATING ___	13 FEARFUL ___	
POUNDING ___	FRIGHTFUL ___	
2 JUMPING ___	TERRIFYING ___	
FLASHING ___	14 PUNISHING ___	
SHOOTING ___	GRUELLING ___	
3 PRICKING ___	CRUEL ___	
BORING ___	VICIOUS ___	
DRILLING ___	KILLING ___	
STABBING ___	15 WRETCHED ___	
LANCINATING ___	BLINDING ___	
4 SHARP ___	16 ANNOYING ___	
CUTTING ___	TROUBLESOME ___	
LACERATING ___	MISERABLE ___	
5 PINCHING ___	INTENSE ___	
PRESSING ___	UNBEARABLE ___	
GNAWING ___	17 SPREADING ___	
CRAMPING ___	RADIATING ___	
CRUSHING ___	PENETRATING ___	
6 TUGGING ___	PIERCING ___	CONSTANT___
PULLING ___	18 TIGHT ___	PERIODIC___
WRENCHING ___	NUMB ___	BRIEF___
7 HOT ___	DRAWING ___	
BURNING ___	SQUEEZING ___	
SCALDING ___	TEARING ___	
SEARING ___	19 COOL ___	

8 TINGLING ___	COLD ___	ACCOMPANYING	SLEEP:	FOOD INTAKE:
ITCHY ___	FREEZING ___	SYMPTOMS:	GOOD ___	GOOD ___
SMARTING ___	20 NAGGING ___	NAUSEA ___	FITFUL ___	SOME ___
STINGING ___	NAUSEATING ___	HEADACHE ___	CAN'T SLEEP ___	LITTLE ___
9 DULL ___	AGONIZING ___	DIZZINESS ___	COMMENTS:	NONE ___
SORE ___	DREADFUL ___	DROWSINESS ___		COMMENTS:
HURTING ___	TORTURING ___	CONSTIPATION ___		
ACHING ___	PPI	DIARRHEA ___		
HEAVY ___	0 No pain ___	COMMENTS:	ACTIVITY:	COMMENTS:
10 TENDER ___	1 MILD ___		GOOD ___	
TAUT ___	2 DISCOMFORTING ___		SOME ___	
RASPING ___	3 DISTRESSING ___		LITTLE ___	
SPLITTING ___	4 HORRIBLE ___		NONE ___	
	5 EXCRUCIATING ___			

213

GLOSSARY

Affective: Relating to the emotions.

Afferent: Conducting inwards; of nerves, towards the brain (cf. *efferent*).

Anaesthesia: Absence of all sensation.

Analgesia: Absence of pain.

Anxiety: A condition of uneasy expectation of harm; it is not the same as fear.

Augmentation-reduction: A bipolar dimension of personality proposed by Asenath Petrie.

Autonomic nervous system: Comprised of the sympathetic and parasympathetic systems (q.v.). Concerned with the regulation of bodily processes relatively independent of the brain.

Axon: That part of a nerve cell forming a nerve fibre conducting impulses *away* from the cell.

Brainstem: The part of the brain lying between the spinal cord and the cerebral cortex.

Central nervous system (CNS): All the nervous tissue comprising the spinal cord and the brain.

Cerebellum: A specialized part of the brain concerned with the integration of muscular movement.

Conditioning: The process of non-cognitive learning, as originally conceived by Pavlov.

Cortex: The outer layer of any organ; the *cerebral cortex* is the uppermost surface of the brain and is concerned with the highest integrative processes.

Cutaneous: Referring to the skin.

Dendrites: Fibres of a nerve cell conducting impulses towards it.

Dorsal: Positioned towards the back.

Dualism: The philosophic view that there is a clear distinction between 'mind' and 'body'.

Efferent: Conducting outwards towards the periphery (cf. *afferent*).

Electromyograph (EMG): A machine that records the varying tensions in muscles.

Electroencephalograph (EEG): A machine that records the varying electrical activity of the brain.

Endorphins: Substances secreted by neural tissue which have a pain-killing action.

Enkephalins: A sub-group of chemicals related to the endorphins, which are secreted in a similar manner.

Evoked potential: An electrical response of the brain to a stimulus, as recorded by appropriate apparatus.

Extraversion: A tendency, presumed to be a fundamental personality trait, to be outgoing, sociable, sensation-seeking and prone to take risks (cf. *introversion*).

Functional disorder: A disorder not clearly due to any tissue damage or cell pathology.

Hypnosis: An artificially-induced state of consciousness, generally held to be characterized by greatly increased suggestibility to the hypnotist.

Hysteria: A type of emotional disorder which has features of histrionic behaviour, sometimes mimicking an organic disorder. The term has no very precise meaning and it tends to be over-used in some branches of psychiatry.

Introversion: The opposite of extraversion (q.v.).

Libido: A term used in psychoanalytic writing to signify a concept of life-energy.

Limbic system: A specialized part of the brain concerned with integrating emotional behaviour.

Motor nerve: A nerve carrying impulses outwards to a muscle or gland.

Mesmerism: The process of inducing a trance state by means that originated with the followers of Mesmer.

Leucotomy: The operation whereby fibres connecting parts of the frontal cortex to lower parts of the brain are severed. (Sometimes called lobotomy.)

Naloxone: A chemical which, when injected into the body, counteracts the effects of morphine and the naturally-occurring endorphins and enkephalins.

Neuron: A nerve cell with all its attached fibres.

Neurophysiology: The scientific study of the physical function of the nervous system.

Neuroticism: A tendency, presumed to be a fundamental personality trait, to be emotionally labile. It is not to be equated with neurotic disorder.

'Noise': The background of irrelevant stimuli (not necessarily of sound) against which we detect those stimuli which are meaningful (q.v. *Sensory Detection Theory*).

Oncologist: A doctor who makes a special study of cancer.

Operant conditioning: The special form of conditioning conceived by B. F. Skinner whereby behaviour is learnt and governed by the consequences of actions.

Opioid: Having an action and chemical nature similar to that of the drugs derived from opium.

Organic disorder: A disorder clearly attributable to damage or physical pathology of the body tissue (cf. *functional disorder*).

Parasympathetic nerves: That part of the autonomic system (q.v.) which promotes resting and recuperative processes.

Peripheral nervous system: All that part of the system lying outside the brain and the spinal cord.

Pineal gland: A small structure in the middle of the brain, of unknown function, which Descartes believed to be the channel of communication between body and soul.

Placebo: From the Latin meaning 'I please'. A substance or procedure that has no intrinsic efficacy, but owes its pain-killing or healing effect to the patient's faith in it.

Psychiatrist: A physician who specializes in the medical aspects of disturbed behaviour.

Psychogenic: Believed to be generated by mental processes.

Psychologist: Someone who has specialized training in the scientific study of behaviour.

Psychophysics: The study of sensory experience in relation to the intensity of the stimulus that produces it.

Reticular formation: That part of the brainstem which is concerned with arousing other parts of the CNS.

Rostral: The front or upper end (literally the 'beak' end).

Sensory Detection Theory (SDT): A theory relating to the perception of events against a background of 'noise' (q.v.). Also known as Signal Detection Theory.

Sensory nerve: A nerve conveying information inwards to the CNS.

Soma: Literally 'the body'. It forms the root of many words.

Sympathetic nerves: That part of the autonomic system (q.v.) which promotes functions concerned with bodily exertion.

Synapse: The communicating junction between two nerve cells.

Thalamus: A brain structure that is largely concerned with linking up different areas by relaying impulses.

Threshold: The lowest point of intensity at which a stimulus is just noticeable.

Ventral: Literally 'to the side of the stomach'; as man stands upright, this means to the front.

Viscera: The organs within the chest and abdomen.

INDEX OF NAMES

Page Numbers in Italics Refer to the References

GENERAL INDEX